Best and Safe Practices in Different Contexts of Neonatal Care

Edited by R. Mauricio Barría

Published in London, United Kingdom

Best and Safe Practices in Different Contexts of Neonatal Care
http://dx.doi.org/10.5772/intechopen.111153
Edited by R. Mauricio Barría

Contributors
Alireza Jashni Motlagh, Amina L. Abubakar, Anjali Tripathy, Annmarie Gennattasio, Azamolmolouk Elsagh, Dagmawit Solomon, Dharmendra Pratap Singh, Dulce Cruz, Enrique Valdés Rubio, Fernando Aguinaga, Firmaye Bogale, Hippolite O. Amadi, Hossam A. Elgnainy, Iosvany Aguiar Ramos, Janet Carvajal de la Osa, Mohammed B. Kawuwa, Mohini Gautam, Osvaldo Flores Belkerbach, Rakesh Dwivedi, Sanskriti Tripathy, Santiago Garzón, Shankar Das, Sovesh Chandra Tripathy, Stephen K. Obaro, Tesfaye Dagne, Tridibesh Tripathy, Vita Boyar, Yenisel Díaz Roller

First published in London, United Kingdom, 2024 by IntechOpen
IntechOpen is the global imprint of INTECHOPEN LIMITED, registered in England and Wales, registration number: 11086078, 167-169 Great Portland Street, London, W1W 5PF, United Kingdom

British Library Cataloguing-in-Publication Data
A catalogue record for this book is available from the British Library

Additional hard and PDF copies can be obtained from orders@intechopen.com

Best and Safe Practices in Different Contexts of Neonatal Care
Edited by R. Mauricio Barría
p. cm.
Print ISBN 978-0-85466-098-8
Online ISBN 978-0-85466-097-1
eBook (PDF) ISBN 978-0-85466-099-5

For EU product safety concerns:
IN TECH d.o.o., Prolaz Marije Krucifikse Kozulić 3, 51000 Rijeka, Croatia,
info@intechopen.com or visit our website at intechopen.com.

Meet the editor

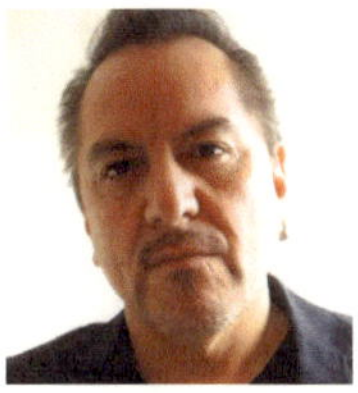

Dr. Mauricio Barría has an Msc and a DrPH in Clinical Epidemiology. He is an associate professor at the Faculty of Medicine, Universidad Austral de Chile, where he has been the creator and director of the Evidence-Based Health Office and the current director of the Institute of Nursing. His areas of undergraduate and graduate teaching and research include maternal–child health, neonatal care, and evidence-based practice. He has conducted numerous research projects and has already published more than seventy articles. Additionally, Dr. Barría is an editorial board member and peer reviewer for journals in nursing, pediatrics, and public health.

Contents

Preface

Neonatal care includes a wide range of interventions and resources needed to provide optimal support for premature and sick newborns, minimize risk, and ensure the highest level of safety. Advances in this field of pediatrics and available evidence have led to the recognition of best practices to implement in a variety of settings and contexts. This book includes important topics related to neonatal care grouped into two sections. In ten chapters addressing relevant topics in neonatal care, the book aims to contribute to the clinical work of healthcare teams in neonatal units.

The initial section is comprised of four chapters that have been developed in a more global manner to analyze the implementation of neonatal care, with a particular focus on the experiences of lower-income countries. Chapter 1, which is based on an analysis of stakeholders and decision-makers in the Ethiopian context, describes the three main issues associated with newborn health, including institutional preparedness and safety, cultural issues, and neonatal care at the policy level. Chapter 2 examines the concepts, characteristics, and constraints related to neonatal care facilities in different regions of Nigeria. It identifies measures to address poor infrastructure in harsh climates and poverty environments in search of designs that enable safe neonatal care and improve the survival of high-risk infants. Chapter 3 presents historical aspects and an analysis of indicators of the current neonatal health situation in India, highlighting a triad of elements of warmth, food, and security care to promote neonatal survival and reduce infant mortality. Chapter 4 reviews the management of outbreaks and infections of multidrug-resistant bacteria in neonatal intensive care units (NICUs), a topic relevant to the neonatal therapeutic environment. It highlights the importance of sanitary and epidemiological surveillance and monitoring interventions.

Section 2 presents essential topics in neonatal care. Chapter 5 describes the issue of noise in neonatal units, and the effects of this exposure on neonates. The analysis explains that understanding modifiable and non-modifiable noise can influence daily practices, NICU design, staff education, and quality improvement programs. Chapter 6 provides background on mechanisms of action, functioning, types, and forms of use of phototherapy in neonates. It also discusses the associated risks and how to address them. Chapters 7 and 8 focus on the prevention and management of pain in the context of care of the critically ill or premature newborn who is exposed to multiple procedures that may generate pain. The chapters highlight interventions or practices that can control or reduce these exposures as well as the painful experience. Chapter 9 addresses the crucial issue of drug safety in neonatal care by considering the neonatal physiology that exposes these patients to increased risks. It discusses high-risk medications and strategies to mitigate these risks. Finally, Chapter 10, through an exhaustive review of the scientific evidence, analyzes the effects of four drugs—aspirin, magnesium sulphate, corticosteroids, and progesterone—on pregnancy and the perinatal period.

As described, this book covers various topics of interest to health professionals involved in neonatal care, emphasizing gathering evidence and experience to implement best practices in the context of patient safety on selected topics. I am grateful to all the authors who, through their contributions from both experience and context, have enabled the development of this interesting book, which should be of use to professionals involved in neonatal care.

R. Mauricio Barría
Institute of Nursing,
Faculty of Medicine,
Universidad Austral de Chile,
Valdivia, Chile

Section 1

Implementation of Neonatal Care in Lower-Income Countries

Chapter 1

Cultural, Institutional and Policy Impact on Neonatal Safety Practice in Ethiopia: A Concept from Policy Dialogue

Tesfaye Dagne, Firmaye Bogale and Dagmawit Solomon

Abstract

The first 28 days is the most critical time for the survival of newborns and is the most essential time to intervene to reduce under-five mortality rapidly. This paper summarized the gaps found related to neonatal mortality in Ethiopia. A stakeholder discussion was held, and a dialogue report was written. From the report, three themes emerged. Institutional level readiness and safety was the first theme where the absence of enough room for neonatal care was stressed. A neonatal intensive care unit is absent in most hospitals. The attention given to neonatal death is minimal compared to labouring mothers. The cultural issue was the second theme in which mourning for the death of a newborn is forbidden. The death of the newborn is handled as a secret, and the burial place is in the backyard. Lastly, the theme of policy-level attention to neonates showed no policy direction guides the audit of neonatal death.

Keywords: child death, dialogue report, Ethiopia, neonatal death, neonatal mortality

1. Introduction

Neonatal mortality is the probability of dying within the first month of life [1, 2]. The first 28 days is the most critical time for the survival of newborns, and it is the most essential time to intervene to reduce under-five mortality too [3] rapidly. Out of the 5.2 million global under-five deaths, about half (2.4 million, 47%) occur among neonates [4, 5].

Almost all neonatal deaths (98%) occur in low- and middle-income countries, with 78% in Southern Asia and sub-Saharan Africa. Eight of the ten countries with the highest neonatal mortality are in Africa including Ethiopia [4–7].

Preterm birth, intrapartum-related complications (birth asphyxia or inability to breathe at birth), infections and congenital disabilities are the main causes of most neonatal mortality [5].

The Sustainable Development Goals (SDG) aimed to reduce neonatal mortality in all countries to at least as low as 12 per 1,000 live births. The 2021 report of SDG shows a global decline of neonatal mortality from 30 to 17 deaths per 1,000 live births [8].

The situation in Ethiopia shows that there was a slow reduction in progress between the years 2000 and 2016, which is a 41% decline when compared to the 60% reduction in under-five mortality and a 50% reduction in infant mortality in the same period [1, 9, 10].

On the other hand, the Ministry of Health of Ethiopia (MoH) planned to reduce neonatal mortality to 21 per 1000 live births at the end of 2024/25 [11]. However, the progress seems to be out of track as the rate of neonatal mortality has shown a rising trend in recent years (from 29 deaths per 1000 live births in 2016 to 33 deaths per 1000 live births in 2019) [1, 10].

Neonatal mortality declined from 46 to 35 deaths per 1000 live births among facility delivery, but the rate remains higher than that of home delivery, which declined from 38 to 30 deaths per 1000 live births. Such higher reports of facility death than that of home delivery were assumed to be associated with the limited service availability and readiness to provide basic essential newborn care services [12].

Thus, these gaps were recognized, and an evidence-based policy brief summarizing the best available evidence to describe the problem of neonatal mortality in Ethiopia and potential solutions for addressing the problem was developed. This evidence-based policy brief was then used to facilitate a stakeholders' dialogue, highlighting and providing insight into the problem itself, its causes, and the solutions indicated in the document. The dialogue participants being from different backgrounds and organizations, the focus of the discussion was multidimensional which touched different aspects of neonatal safety and care. The cultural influence and aspect of neonatal mortality are stressed during the dialogue. The emphasis given to neonatal health issues at policy level, institutional/health facility level and societal/community level was also raised. These entail practice, safety, perception and national direction surrounding neonatal health. Hence, the authors of the evidence-based policy brief tried to summarize the idea of the dialogue participants in a structured manner so that it will be an input for policymakers, programme managers, healthcare professionals, partners working on reducing neonatal mortality and any interested stakeholders. This concept paper tried to bring comprehensive factors that are critical in improving the health of neonates.

So, the concept paper is significant for policymakers, programme managers, clinicians and other health professionals in identifying the gaps found in the health and safety of neonates. The paper also shows a fertile area where researchers can embark in the future by bringing new findings and recommendations. Moreover, this paper tried to look at the most widely overrun issue of neonatal care and safety and cultural issues that influence neonatal health. In general, this paper is expected to provide critical insight into the future of neonatal care and policy in Ethiopia.

2. Methods

A structured discussion focused on an evidence-based policy brief was held in Ethiopia for 2 days by participating key stakeholders working on neonatal health. This discussion, namely "stakeholders' dialogue on Reducing Neonatal Mortality in Ethiopia: A Call for Urgent Action!" served as a scientific discussion platform to get and incorporate constructive evidence into a document that was produced by researchers and helped enrich the evidence-based policy brief document with more insights to inform policymakers.

The dialogue was prepared by the knowledge translation directorate at the Ethiopian Public Health Institute. This brief was prepared by a team composed of experts on evidence synthesis from the knowledge translation directorate of the Ethiopian Public Health Institute and experts on neonatal health from the Federal Ministry of Health of Ethiopia.

The dialogue was held in May 2021 for 2 days. Brief sensitization presentations on knowledge translation and health technology assessment and presentation on the prepared evidence-based policy brief were made and discussions were held. The discussions reflected on neonatal mortality with the community/societal perception of neonatal death, the facility level attention and the policy level attention given to neonatal death.

The dialogue report was translated into English and written verbatim from the note of note-takers (six note-takers). Then, based on the content of the dialogue report, thematization was carried out. Accordingly, cultural issues, institutional issues and policy-level issues were identified as three themes that emerged from the dialogue report. So, we prepared this paper based on the discussion output from different professionals, representatives, and governmental and non-governmental organizations.

2.1 Method of discussion

The policy brief document prepared by the knowledge translation team of the Ethiopian Public Health Institute (EPHI) on "Reducing Neonatal Mortality" was provided to each participant to go through the document. Then, the discussion was moderated by an experienced professor. The following rules were applied during the discussion:

- Every participant has an equal right to participate and contribute in the dialogue regardless of his/her position or the organization he/she is delegated from.
- The dialogue does not NECESSARILY aim for consensus rather, it aims to generate insight and perspectives on the issues.
- The participants should choose language for discussion; feel free to express your opinion in a language you prefer to do so.
- Chatham House Rule, which states that: "Participants are free to use the information received during the meeting, but neither the identity nor the affiliation of the speaker(s), nor that of any other participant, may be revealed," should respected.

2.2 Participant of the dialogue

About 50 invited professionals and non-professionals from different organization participated in the meeting. Participants were invited from governmental organizations (federal, regional, zonal and district representatives), specialized hospitals which mainly focus on neonatal care, non-governmental organizations working on neonatal programmes, community representatives, the House of People's Representatives and the Office of the Prime Minister. Professionally, participants were neonatologists, public health professionals, health extension workers (community health workers from rural and urban), clinicians, researchers, consultants, programme managers, policymakers, etc.

3. Discussion outputs

3.1 Facility-level attention to neonatal death and safety of care

The safety of care provided for neonates at the health facility level is questionable in Ethiopia. The dialogue participants stressed that there were not enough rooms for neonatal care at health facilities as all attention is given exclusively to the labouring mother during delivery. This is because maternal death is given much attention at the national level and brings accountability for incidents. A neonatal intensive care unit (NICU) is absent in most hospitals, and the available units are just for name-holding with minimum functionality. Most NICU rooms lack the necessary materials, professionals and other supplies. The location of the NICU room is usually at some corner of the corridor of hospitals with minimal space.

When a pregnant mother comes to the hospital for delivery, there will be a gynecologist, obstetrician, midwifery and other professionals for the mother. The room is equipped in a way that will support the mother during labour and birth. But in most cases, no professional is just committed to caring for the newborn. There is no pediatrician or neonatologist in the room.

The location of the neonatal room is another problem. As discussed earlier, the room committed for neonatal care is at some corner of a hospital building and is usually too far away from the delivery room. It puts newborns at risk of exposure to uncontrolled temperature when transporting them to the other room. This is worsened by a structural problem. Delivery room and neonatal room should be designed in a way that it could keep both the mother and newborn safe, which is not common here since most hospitals are initially designed without a neonatal room, and the rooms are added later to accompany the need for neonatal care now.

Whenever there is a maternal death, there will be a shock wave across the health institute where the death happened, there will be an investigation for the cause of the death, and higher officials will be part of the team to identify the cause of death and try to bring accountability. But when there is death of neonates, in most cases, nobody in the hospital and higher officials are concerned. It is common to hear such cases, and nobody is in a position to investigate the cause of death. Sometimes, the death of a newborn is reported as a stillbirth at hospitals, not to take responsibility for the death by health professionals. Such practice has the probability of under-reporting the rate of neonatal mortality in the country, suppressing the search for a solution to the problem.

A clear indication of less emphasis on the death of neonates is seen by the fact that every hospital has a team assigned to investigate the cause of every maternal death, which does not hold for neonatal death. The team is there to exhaustively analyze the cause of maternal mortality and provide a full investigation report to the next higher level. This allows the higher level to analyze the cause, categorize the issue, give feedback to the lower level, and take corrective actions.

3.2 Policy level attention to neonates and adapting best practice

As mentioned in the introductory part, reducing neonatal and maternal deaths is the top priority area of low- and middle-income countries. It is also among the global agendas. But the attention given to these two areas of priority is not uniform. Although there is a strategy for child survival, it is indicated by the dialogue

DOI: http://dx.doi.org/10.5772/intechopen.1003120

participants that there is no guideline to investigate neonatal death as "There is guideline that guide the activity of practitioners to investigate and report the case of maternal death. There is a system called Maternal Death Surveillance and Report (MDSR). But, unlike the death of mothers there are no developed guidelines that help investigate the death of neonates. There is no policy direction that guide the audit and investigation of neonatal death."

In Ethiopia, there was a movement called "No mother should die while giving birthlife," to raise community awareness and funds for activities to reduce maternal mortality. After the initiative was started, the community and government purchased different resources like ambulances, which were committed to serving pregnant mothers. Community awareness was also focused on reducing maternal death through media, community education and other means. This initiative successfully created awareness and sensitized the community on maternal death. Unfortunately, similar or comparable initiatives are not in place to address neonatal deaths like maternal deaths. Thus, it is recommended that a direction for the future could be adapting and piloting similar initiatives and movements that have been seen to be effective in reducing maternal death burden and bringing awareness around neonatal mortality.

3.3 Community/societal perception of neonatal death

> *There is a perception by the community that newborns are not considered as human beings. Even their death is not recognized as human death but simply as material loss referred as 'it disappeared' or 'Tefa/ጠፋ' in Amharic language and only a mother mourns the death of her neonate baby to whom the loss is real.*

Culturally, it is forbidden to mourn for the death of a newborn because newborns are not considered human. There will be no tent erected for the death of a newborn like how it is done for any other person. The death of newborn is handled as a secret, and the burial place is in the backyard. But the burial place for any older individual is in a proper graveyard in a church or a selected place. There will be few or no gatherings of families, community and relatives for the death of the newborn. In most cases, the death of newborn is not announced to relatives and neighbors. But older people's death is usually given much attention and is accompanied by many ceremonies. For the death of the old, families and relatives will be informed of the death, people will have waited to join the burial ceremony for days, and there will be a big gathering during the burial day. But for the newborn who has not started life and is not a full being yet, as the common saying goes in society, there is nothing to be done for his/her death.

Different signs are non-verbal representations of someone who has lost a close person in Ethiopia. These include making a tent in front of the home of the family of deceased, wearing black cloth, not shaving hair and beard (for males), not wearing beautifying ornaments, not using different make-ups for beautifying, etc. This norm, however, is neglected and sometimes seen as inappropriate when it comes to the death of a neonate.

4. Discussion

This concept paper was prepared to capture the pertinent points from the dialogue conducted on the evidence brief prepared on the reduction of neonatal mortality in

Ethiopia. Hence, the outputs of the discussion were summarized and presented in three themes. These are institutional issues, policy-level issues and cultural issues.

Looking at institutional issues related with neonatal care, it is indicated that hospitals and other health facilities are not well equipped and safe to provide effective service to neonates. The attention given to neonates at health facilities is sub-optimal compared to the magnitude of the problem. The dialogue participants emphasized the negligence of neonatal services at health facilities compared to other services. This claim was supported by a survey that assessed the readiness of more than 100 primary hospitals in Ethiopia. The survey reported that the minimum national neonatal intensive care unit (NICU) standard requirement for infrastructure was met by only 63% of hospitals. The average number of neonatal intensive care unit-trained nurses per primary hospital was below the recommended national standard. The survey also found that the minimum national requirement for medical equipment and renewables for neonate care was met only by 24% hospitals, 65% for essential laboratory tests, and 87% for clinical services and procedures [13].

On the other hand, neonatal care during birth is given less attention at health facilities in Ethiopia, especially during birth. While everybody rushes to save the lives of the mother, neonates get neglected. Different professionals are assigned to attend delivery, but no specialized professional is assigned for neonatal care during birth. Report finding also shows that about 61% of neonatal death is accounted to poor quality of care, and only about half of maternal death is associated with poor quality of care [14].

Neonatal death is also not well counted and reported as it happens. Most of the time, neonatal death is counted and recorded as still birth. Different documents also discuss the problem of undercounting and under-reporting neonatal deaths, which in turn is a critical problem in identifying the cause of deaths and devising effective interventions [2, 5].

In Ethiopia, there was an impactful policy attention/movement on the reduction of maternal mortality. There was a visible commitment from policymakers and programme managers to the movement. This can be evidenced by the conferences being held here and there with the motto of "No woman should die while giving life," which mainly focused on the mother, not the newborn [15, 16]. There were regular women/pregnant mother conferences and gatherings aimed to improve mother awareness of institutional delivery led by health professionals. At such conferences, the major topic discussed was institutional delivery, where neonatal mortality or safety was bypassed. Such important initiatives and attention should have also been given to neonatal care. Nevertheless, there is no such initiative that focuses on neonatal mortality.

There is a system of auditing, investigating and reporting maternal deaths in Ethiopia. Guidelines were developed, and training was also provided to health professionals working on maternal health. The guideline is a way of finding the number of mother who died during delivery, where they died and the reason for their death [17, 18]. But, no such system exists to record and study the reason for newborn death. This clearly manifests the political commitment to maternal health and sub-optimal attention to neonatal mortality. Therefore, given that the attention provided to maternal health is encouraging, similar initiatives should be expanded to care for newborns.

At the community level, the death of a newborn is not considered the death of a human being. It is kept a secret and is not known to neighbors, relatives or others. The burial process is commonly managed by the birth attendant (usually grandmothers, older women or traditional birth attendants). These practices and perceptions were confirmed by a study conducted in Ethiopia. According to the study, neonates are considered "strangers to families and neighbours" because newborns are unknown to neighbors or relatives. The study states that if a newborn is dead after birth, it is not treated as human by the culture of the society. The participants replied that mourning for the death of a newborn is not culturally acceptable. Even mourning for a newborn is considered as if it brings more bad incidents like additional death to the family [9, 19]. The burial process of a deceased newborn is in the home of the family or in the backyard, which is done with an intent to keep the death hidden. The burial process is only known to family members, few relatives and close neighbors [19].

5. Implications and recommendations

The community-level perception of the death of newborns can impact reducing the death of neonatal mortality. Such type of practice in society makes the death of newborns get less attention from decision makers, policymakers and programme managers. It also masks the investigation of the cause of neonatal death and leaves neonatal death uncounted because neonatal death remains hidden in society. So, neonatal mortality should be made public and discussed so that possible solutions can be sought at community, facility or policy level.

At the health facility, again, minimal attention was given to the death of neonates. All attention is on saving the mother, especially during labour and birth. Even though this is a positive practice, it should not be done at the expense of neonatal care, as this is a critical time to save the lives of many neonates. There is structural or institutional marginalization of neonates at the health facility level. Such marginalization of neonatal care at health facilities should be intervened by programme managers, policymakers and health professionals. As gynecologists, obstetricians and midwives are assigned to attend delivery and care for the mother, neonatologist, pediatrician or neonatal nurses should accompany the newborn to the labour ward.

There should be a system of auditing and reporting neonatal deaths so that possible interventions can be made. A team or committee that works on neonatal mortality should be established at every health facility, such as the Maternal Death Surveillance and Report (MDSR). It should be noted that improving the system of reporting neonatal mortality is a matter of human right and a means of reducing neonatal mortality.

At a policy level, even though there are guidelines and initiatives, neonatal mortality is not given due attention despite the scale of the problem. Guidelines and directives should be developed for safer neonatal care and properly reporting and counting neonatal mortality. Like that of maternal death, similar initiatives and movements should be in place to advocate for and create community awareness on the issue of neonatal safety and mortality.

To sum up, all actors including community members, policymakers and health professionals, should look at the existing gaps and work collaboratively to reverse the current trend of neonatal mortality. There should be initiatives and a supportive policy environment to support advocacy of neonatal care. The impactful initiatives implemented to reduce maternal mortality in Ethiopia should be expanded for neonatal health and safety. There should be platforms to transfer knowledge from effective interventions in other areas, like maternal care, to neonatal care. Health facilities' wards and departments should be redesigned in a way that can enhance the health and safety of neonates.

Authors' contributions

All authors equally participated in organizing the dialogue meeting. Throughout the entire event, all authors took notes. All authors wrote the final document after discussing the paper's subject, structure and concept. The final text was revised and approved by all authors. The final document was read and approved by the author(s).

Funding

The dialogue meeting was organized with the support of the Partnership for Evidence and Equity in Responsive Social Systems (PEERSS). There is no funding obtained for the preparation and publication of this specific manuscript.

Competing interests

The authors declare that they have no competing interests.

Author details

Tesfaye Dagne*, Firmaye Bogale and Dagmawit Solomon
Knowledge Translation Directorate, Ethiopian Public Health Institute, Addis Ababa, Ethiopia

*Address all correspondence to: tesfayedagne6@gmail.com

References

[1] Federal Democratic Republic of Ethiopia. Maryland, USA: ICF Rockville; 2016

[2] WHO. Making every baby count: Audit and review of stillbirths and neonatal deaths. WHO Library Catalysis Data. 2016;**2016**:144

[3] UNICEF. Committing to child survival: A promise renewed. [Online]. 2014. Available from: http://www.unicef.fr/userfiles/UNICEF_Progress_Report_2012_Child-survival.pdf

[4] UNICEF and WHO. Survive and thrive – Transforming care for every small and sick newborn: Key findings. 2020; p. 10

[5] WHO. Newborn mortality. Key Facts; 2022. Available from: https://www.who.int/news-room/fact-sheets/detail/levels-and-trends-in-child-mortality-report-2021

[6] UN Inter-agency Group for Child Mortality Estimation, UNICEF, WHO, and WBO. Levels & trends in child mortality estimation child mortality. [Online]. 2020. Available from: https://www.unicef.org/media/79371/file/UN-IGME-child-mortality-report-2020.pdf

[7] United Nations. The 2030 agenda and the sustainable development goals an opportunity for Latin America and the Caribbean Thank you for your interest in this ECLAC publication. 2018

[8] United Nations. The sustainable development goals report 2021. United Nations Public. Issued by Department of Economic and Social Affairs. 2021; 1-64

[9] MoH. National Reproductive Health Strategy, 2016 – 2020. [Online]. 2016. Available from: https://www.usaid.gov/sites/default/files/documents/1860/EthiopiaDHS2016KIR-final10-17-2016.pdf

[10] Federal Democratic Republic of Ethiopia. Maryland, USA: ICF Rockville; 2019

[11] FMoH. Health Sector Transformation Plan (HSTP-II) 2020/21-2024/25 (2013 EFY–2017 EFY). 2021

[12] F. M. of H. and E. P. H. Institute. Understanding the derivers of reduction in maternal and neonatal mortality in Ethiopia- An in-depth case study of Global Exemplers. 2022

[13] Abawollo HS, Tsegaye ZT, Desta BF, Beshir IA. Readiness of primary hospitals in providing neonatal intensive Care Services in Ethiopia. Ethiopian Journal of Health Sciences. 2021;**31**(2):321-328. DOI: 10.4314/ejhs.v31i2.15

[14] WHO & UNICEF. The every new born action plan: Ending preventable newborn deaths and stillbirths by 2030. [Online]. 2020. Available from: https://www.unicef.org/media/77166/file/Ending-preventable-newborn-deaths-and-stillbirths-by-2030-universal-health-coverage-in-2020-2025.pdf

[15] WHO. No woman should die while giving life: Safe motherhood month calls for zero home deliveries. 2015. Available from: https://www.afro.who.int/news/no-woman-should-die-while-giving-life-safe-motherhood-month-calls-zero-home-deliveries

[16] World Vision. Practicing faith. Four stories from Ethiopia, engaging faith leaders for better maternal health. 2015

[17] MoH. Maternal death surveillance and response (MDSR) technical guideline. 2012

[18] I. C. of M. FIGO, UKaid, E4A, UNFPA, CDC, WHO. Maternal death surveillance and report. Technical guidance. Information for action to prevent maternal death. 2013

[19] Sisay MM, Yirgu R, Gobezayehu AG, Sibley LM. A qualitative study of attitudes and values surrounding stillbirth and neonatal mortality among grandmothers, mothers, and unmarried girls in rural Amhara and Oromiya regions, Ethiopia: Unheard souls in the backyard. Journal of Midwifery Women's Health. 2014;**59**(Suppl. 1). DOI: 10.1111/jmwh.12156

Chapter 2

Fundamentals of a Safe and Effective Neonatal Building Design in a Tropical Low-Income Setting

Hippolite O. Amadi, Mohammed B. Kawuwa,
Amina L. Abubakar and Stephen K. Obaro

Abstract

A safe and effective neonatal building is an aspect of Neonatal Rescue Scheme (NRS) concept as described in the literature. Observable habitual practices leading to various neonatal outcomes at tropical LMIC settings point to adverse facility-based mortality contributions from poor nursery layouts. Sadly, the negative impacts of building deficiencies are not well-understood or empirically quantified as tailored to the limitations in resource-constrained tropical climate. Lack of helpful building features may exacerbate high morbidity owing to adverse issues such as poor infection control, evening fever syndrome (EFS), noise pollution, medication safety, intra-ward traffic, nursing fatigue, and parental services. A tropical LMIC setting has the disadvantages of relative poverty, infrastructural inadequacies, and adverse equatorial climatic conditions, necessitating design-specific requirements for safe neonatal care. This chapter is proposed to explore the constraints, concepts, and features as integrated in some NRS nurseries at different tropical regions of Nigeria, which function to mitigate the climate, poor infrastructure, and societal poverty against neonatal survival.

Keywords: neonatal mortality, tropical LMIC, nursery building, neonatal rescue scheme, climate change

1. Introduction

The low- and middle-income countries (LMICs) of the world, particularly in Africa, are riddled with so many disadvantages emanating from poverty and lack of basic infrastructure for effective neonatal care. The lack of these basic neonatal practice needs, in turn, exposes the neonate to unimaginable hardships and unsafe environments in their struggle for survival. Literature is dominated by research, discoveries, advances in practices, methodologies, and technologies showcasing neonatal care in high-income countries (HICs) of the world. The attractive technologies and highly successful neonatal outcomes at HICs are made possible by highly sustainable funding and infrastructure, which are readily available to practitioners at HICs, the very opposite of the situations at LMICs. Whenever a typical practitioner at an LMIC setting searches the literature for new ideas to better practice, swarms of articles of HIC technologies and ideas would dominate the horizon, compelling the practitioner to gravitate to these ideas as the best that could be used. LMIC practitioners very often forget that all successes at HICs are fundamentally made possible by the sustainable infrastructure that creates the conducive environments and climate which helps the technologies to thrive and produce attractive results. Consequently, the LMIC practitioners need to be articulative and consciously understand that a rush into the adoption of many of these HIC technologies and ideas without initiation of commensurate sustainable funding and infrastructure would always amount to neonatal practice suicide. We hypothesize that lack of conscious understanding and reaction to this very situation of impoverishment is the backdrop of the perpetual high neonatal mortality rate at most LMIC settings, including Nigeria.

The advantages created by the opportunity of simultaneously being a senior medical professional at a top HIC institution as well as a visiting consultant at many top LMIC hospitals have enabled this corresponding author to amass a vast amount of experience to respond to the disadvantages of the LMIC settings. Therefore, it is essential to note that this LMIC ugly situation can be intelligently divided into two segments, which must be recognized and treated with prioritization. Hence, if an LMIC setting must successfully adopt the HIC, then it is necessarily required to proceed as follows: (1) The LMIC setting must put in place a good quality and sustainable infrastructure like power, access road, and sustainable treatment funding that is tailored after those in HIC settings, after which (2) The LMIC facility could proceed to adopt the efficient new ideas and technologies tailored after those in HIC settings. The LMIC governments and their neonatal practitioners who are often drawn to the HIC high-tech, without prioritizing their infrastructural base, would always end up in unsustainable outcomes and the re-emergence of facility failures that were once thought to have been resolved. However, in situations where the government and in-country policy makers fail to understand these arguments, then the practitioners and local facility management must come to the rescue of the endangered neonate by adopting other strategies at their disposal. Hospital management may be unable to bypass the government to build sustainable grid electric supply, good access roads and highway network, and prosperous economy for neonatal carers. However, they are certainly capable of ingeniously creating facility buildings, and onsite harnessing and exploitation of nature as a response to the adverse neonatal effects of government failures. Better survival rate of neonates using alternative ingenious techniques which did not rely on standard government-led infrastructure have previously been demonstrated [1–4].

Neonates at LMIC facilities are notably exposed to all kinds of unsafe situations that threaten them with immediate death or later life disabilities. Many of the health threats can be avoided by designing and adopting some possible facility building features. However, these features can only be conceptualized with a good understanding of what these neonatal unsafe situations really represent. Neonatal facility buildings are erroneously, not often regarded as one of the most sensitive neonatal equipment that must not be compromised. Therefore, these buildings have been designed and constructed without any reference to the deadly dangers and unsafe environment the nursery building would present to the neonates. The deadly mistake of this ignorance has exacerbated the negative impacts of morbidities that neonates would have to deal with, hence, making many of them to easily lose their battles for survival. A nursery building that incorporates adequate responses to neonatal adverse effects and conditions is termed a 'functional building'. A nursery building that exacerbates the negative climatic, economic, and socio-cultural effects is a 'dysfunctional building'. Therefore, a knowledgeably designed nursery building can mitigate the effects of adverse climate, technology and policy-failures, socio-cultural dispositions, carer poverty, and lack of essential social infrastructure.

This chapter will explore a few of the neonatal unsafe conditions as have been identified across the entire regions of Nigeria, and the implemented nursery building designs and features that have been used to mitigate their impacts on neonatal survival.

2. Building with intent to shield neonates against hyperthermia

Sub-Saharan Africa is notable for high sunlight intensity for almost every month of the year, with some regions recording outdoor temperatures higher than 46°C and spanning many hours of the day [5]. The consequent high indoor nursery temperature has, for many years, been responsible for misdiagnoses of the iatrogenic fever as a disease-process requiring antibiotic intervention, from which neonates have lost their lives [5]. However, this climate-induced evening fever syndrome (EFS) would normally wear-off much later in the night or with the relocation of the neonate to a cooler spot within the nursery space, and without the need of antibiotics as has been demonstrated in the literature [5, 6]. The deadly effects of EFS could be avoided if the choice of the site and positioning of the nursery apartment within the neonatal building complex is made with full evaluation of the predictable interactions and impacts of light rays as the sun rises from the eastern cardinal direction and sets at the western. The neglect or ignorance of EFS mitigation would lead to daily neonatal hyperthermia, complications from needlessly administered antibiotics, and neonatal thermal-shock from practices that attempt to rapidly force-down the body temperature, which could lead to death [7].

Unprotected sunrays interactions with nursery interiors have many other negative impacts on the workforce, including staff discomfort and tiredness. Since the neonates experiencing hyperthermia would not be left unattended, the nursing staff must expend extra labour in trying whatever possible to keep the neonates safe. This situation is made worse during occasions when many neonates are overpowered by EFS effects, simultaneously. Unfortunately, lack of adequate nursing manpower in a typical special care baby unit (SCBU) is an endemic LMIC situation [8]. Therefore, dysfunctional nursery apartments at LMICs, where there may not be sustainable luxuries of electric powered air-conditioning systems, create a wide variety of practice difficulties and unsafe environment for the neonate. Naturally cooled nursery environment at such high intensity sunny settings help to ensure conducive thermal tranquility for neonates and the staff who look after them. Therefore, features of 'double-wall, air-lagged' techniques, and SCBU-floor underground lowering, as described in the literature has been adopted in some recent SCBU buildings in Nigeria (**Figure 1**).

3. Building with intent to enhance low-cost facility lighting and power supply

Inadequate and erratic power supply has been blamed amongst other factors responsible for high mortality at LMIC health facilities [9]. The health facilities in Nigeria are notoriously crippled by incessant power blackouts, including at high

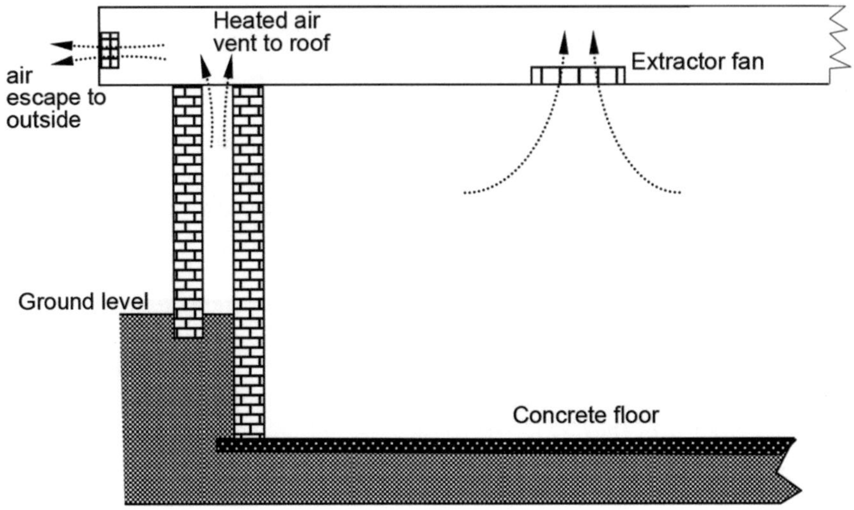

Figure 1.
Air-lagged double wall technique as described in Amadi et al. [5].

vulnerability hospital segments such as the SCBU [10]. Hence, some useful methods of alternative or supplementary power provision have been suggested, including the use of solar panels and inverter technology [11]. The conventional technique of inverter power installation in Nigeria involves connection of the panel-battery-inverter assembly as a standby power supplier in the event of grid power failure. This technique has limitations that often create practice frustrations as has been observed across many Nigerian SCBUs applying this. Some centres have explained their frustrations for the lack of sustainability of this power option, including the high cost of frequent battery replacement. Other centres complained of the short lifespan of the standby inverter power supply after full charge, which could only support facility lighting and powering the essential neonatal machines at night for less than 3 h before the SCBU returned to utter blackout for the rest of the night. There are explainable technical reasons for this short lifespan, including inefficiency of the installation technique that are often applied. The separation of the duo of 'facility lighting' and 'sockets powering' into two independent systems when using renewable energy backup has previously been proposed [2]. The proposal demonstrated how the Neonatal Unit could be powered by two independent solar panel gangs, one supplying 12 V to its charge controllers and the other supplying 48 V, respectively. Therefore, nursery building design and construction must create adequate provision for the components that could be later installed for this purpose, such as various gangs of roof-mounted solar panels and rooftop wind breakers for panel protection (**Figure 2**).

3.1 Independent lighting system

Conventionally, the inverter power is typically wired into the existing nursery power distribution lines using 'switchover gear' controls via chosen fuse-lines. Using this technique, specific fuse-lines for power sockets and gangs of lighting points are selected to be supplied by the inverter. This measure is a power management technique to restrict the standby inverter power to the relevant sections of the nursery, where all the conventional high voltage outputs along the prioritized lines are

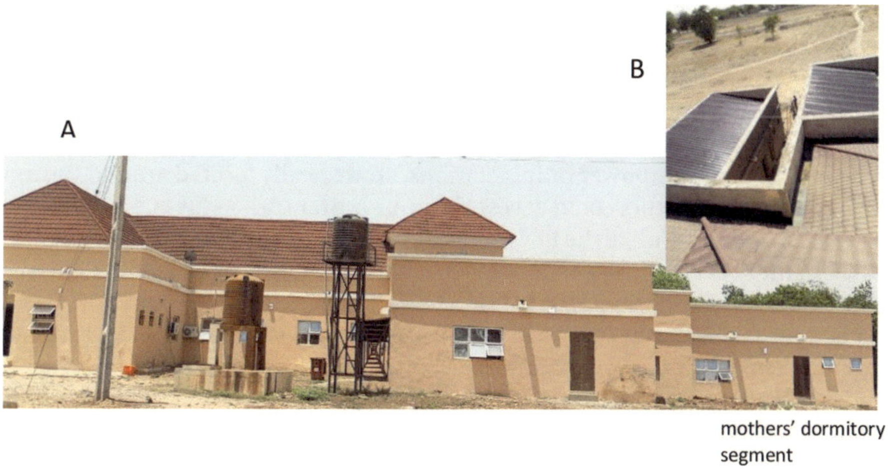

Figure 2.
(A) Sideview Yobe NRS neonatal hubcentre complex (B) Part of rooftop – mothers' dormitory segment – showing roof wind breaker parapet before solar panel installation.

enabled. Therefore, the inverter system is subjected to supply energy to all conventional light bulbs, some of which could be of high-power consumption ratings, such as 60–100 W, as often installed in a typical SCBU in Nigeria. It has been previously reported that the inverter system installed in this manner would readily get drained of its battery reserve in quick time, leading to automatic self 'power off'. The use of low wattage bulbs, such as 5–12 W, had been tried but this did not yield much overall improvement. Also, illumination from the low wattage bulbs was described as insufficient in intensity for some aspects of clinical works, such as 'neonatal line-setting' in the night. Amadi and Abubakar [2] demonstrated their 'polite-light-bank (PLB)' system, which was a successful response to the need of making the solar power backup to sufficiently last an entire night with high intensity of illumination throughout. The PLB was a separate low voltage wiring independently distributed across the walkways and rooms of the nursery building. Hence, the lighting system so-demonstrated was a standalone 12 V system, which relieved the inverter system from the power-draining light bulbs. The application of the PLB technology as an essential system for an LMIC neonatal unit would require that a standard nursery building construction is strategically integrated with features for seamless installation of the PLB technology.

3.2 Individualized power buffer station

Modern day neonatology is highly reliant on machines and gadgets that are electrically powered. Experience from notable Neonatal Units in Nigeria, such as the Amina-centre in Minna and the Neoroom at CWCH Calabar, have shown that the application of the PLB enabled their standby power bank systems to sustain all power sockets longer than 12 h, covering the entire night hours of work [2]. However, this time coverage can easily drop by half during full unit capacity when many power-guzzling systems could be working simultaneously. A centre could have up to four oxygen concentrators, ten incubators, eight phototherapy machines, four ventilators, infusion pumps, and other life-support gadgets running at the same time. Our LMIC neonatal research efforts have strived to develop assembles of systems that could generate, store, and manage solar power for dusk-to-dawn facility energy supply to sustain facility operations until sunrise of the next day, when the batteries begin to re-charge again. Hence, our recent research has focused on the creation of an effective technical response to this scenario of 'full house' power demand to ensure all-night power coverage. The individualized power buffer station was, hence, conceptualized. In our concept, a typical 20 cot/incubator space capacity neonatal nursery is designed with a minimum of four power buffer stations, strategically located around the inner ward where two incubators could access the same buffer station for energy without being moved around. Unlike the main central powerbank system which is fully installed in the separate power room of the nursery complex, an individual buffer-station is located within the ward. This is a brick-built enclosure (length 600 mm, width 600 mm, height 300 mm) with ventilation openings on the sides and strongly secured wooden top cover. Each buffer-station is equipped with two numbers of 12 V, 150AH batteries connected in parallel, linked to the 12 V panel gang supply and recharged via a dedicated MTTP charge-controller. The buffer-station delivers outputs of 12 V DC via cigarette lighter sockets (**Figure 3**), and 230 V AC via a dedicated 3.0 KVA inverter.

4. Building with intent to enhance nursing supervision

Shortage of nursing staff and poor nursing management techniques have all been previously associated with the factors identified to exacerbate high neonatal mortality in Nigeria [8, 12]. Amadi et al. [13] emphasized the need for LMIC facilities to improve on their staff strengths for their ever-busy neonatal centres, citing the Nigerian poor situation where the ratio of nurses-to-neonates per duty-shift was 1:10, or something worse. This poor ratio is not getting any better as the devastating economic situation in these countries has further fueled the massive exodus of qualified nurses out of the countries in search of better-paid jobs in foreign lands,

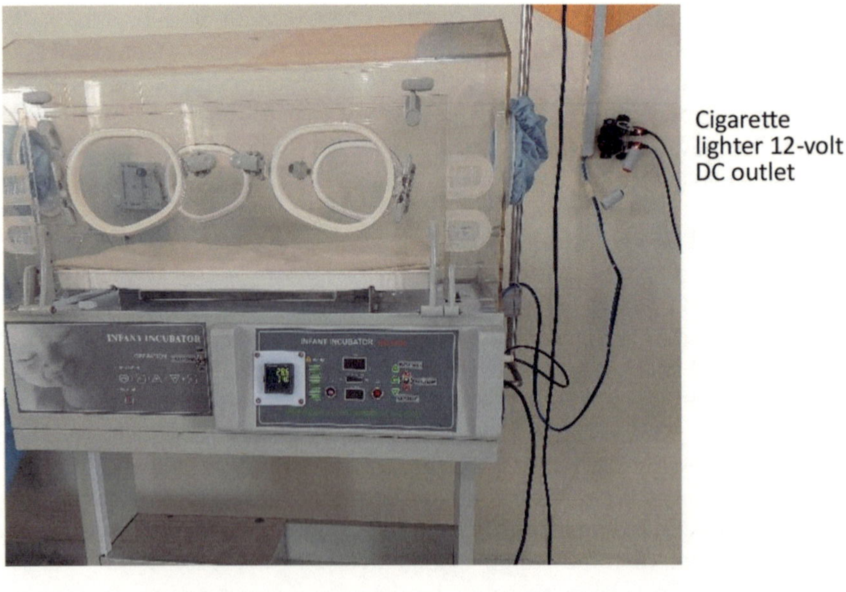

Figure 3.
Cigarette lighter output at a buffer-station at SCBU-1 of the Federal Medical Centre, Owerri.

particularly in the HICs. It has, therefore, become more difficult to stop or limit the Nursing Management of hospitals from their incessant staff-reshuffling, which leads to the posting of inexperienced nurses to work at the neonatal wards [13]. The exodus of experienced nurses has also resulted in a massive shortage of capable supervisors to guide the growing numbers of young or inexperienced nurses to whom the poor neonates are exposed in their on-the-job trial and error learning technique. The changing dynamics and SCBU nurses' demography present the need for radical responses to counter the effects from any alterable avenues.

Typical, the Nigerian SCBU operations vests a lot of administrative duties on the Head Nurse (sometimes called the in-charge, chief-matron, or ward-manager), often keeping this senior staff away from the routine nursing work. SCBU-building segments in Nigeria are usually incorporated with ward-manager's office, which are located away from the neonatal nursery halls. Head-nurses are unable to observe an on-going error in real-time for immediate intervention unless these happen during the few occasions when the head-nurse finds the time to walk into the hall for a quick look-around. Neonatal head-nurses could multitask the demanding administrative work with real-time nurses' supervision to minimize fatal errors as has been orchestrated by the shortage of experienced neonatal nurses. This challenge, hence, inspired the new concept of creating nursery buildings that enhance the opportunity for head-nurses to multitask.

The new concept as has been implemented by our team ensures that the head-nurses' office shares a common wall with the main nursery hall of the complex, such that the head-nurse is allowed a controllable panoramic view of all the work areas from the comfort of the managerial office. The adjoining walls could be developed into large see-through interactive windows and communication ports to aid the views of the manager and the ability to offer real-time instructions during work (**Figure 4**).

5. Building-features with intent to enhance low-cost oxygen availability

Our on-the-job experience shows that piped-oxygen systems are too expensive to acquire and install at the resource constrained settings we assessed. However, the few hospitals that managed to procure and set up the oxygen system could not sustain these, and soon abandoned the use of the system due to high operational costs. Therefore, we conclude that many adverse factors make the imported brands of the technology unsustainable, even at the moderately well-to-do places of the LMICs [3].

One of the neonatal healthcare limitations of hinterland LMICs is unsustainable access to adequate supply of oxygen for neonatal respiratory support. Respiratory distress is a common condition that presents in very-low preterm or extremely-low birthweight neonates. Premature neonates who are born in the hinterlands are, by default, left to faith for survival as most attempts to access specialist care in the city are usually unsuccessful due to the often-treacherous transportation methods used. Neonatal lives can be easily saved if local healthcare Centre practitioners are trained in simple mechanized assistive breathing techniques. However, one of the major impediments would remain source-able oxygen for the mechanized applications. This chapter has already explored and presented ideas of sustainable generation, storage, and management of solar-harnessed power for usage at these remote locations of the world. We have used such energy to directly operate low-voltage (12 V DC) oxygen concentrators that produce up to 5 LPM oxygen flow, as this technology is commonly available in the

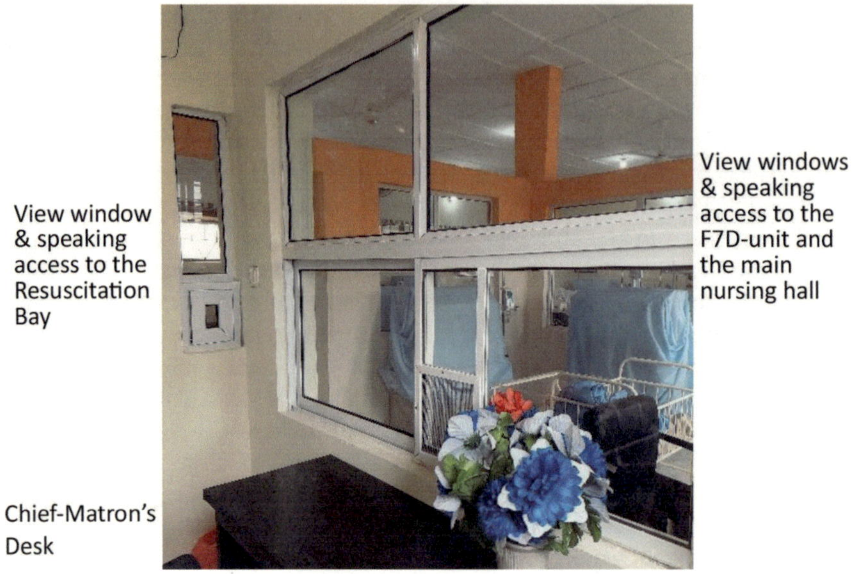
View window & speaking access to the Resuscitation Bay
View windows & speaking access to the F7D-unit and the main nursing hall
Chief-Matron's Desk

Figure 4.
Ward manager's office at SCBU-1 of the Federal Medical Centre (FMC), Owerri.

internet market. At some of our centres, we use inverted high-voltage (220 V AC) from our battery storage to operate higher-power oxygen concentrators producing 8–10 LPM of oxygen flow. These technologies for real-time oxygen production at remote locations can be easily assembled. However, the high-power consumption rate of the compressors that operate the concentrators makes it difficult to run more than one or two such machines, simultaneously, without a quick depletion of the limited energy storage. This problem inspired our recent research to develop a low-cost sustainable method of distributing the generated oxygen to reach multiple patients, simultaneously. This is our 'politeoxygen splitter system (the PSS)' technology [3].

The PSS is capable of sharing and delivering the output from a single oxygen concentrator to reach up to eight neonates with patient-specific controls of prescribed individual flowrates simultaneously. This makes the PSS an essential feature of an NRS neonatal building design, within the cities and rural places of Nigeria. Therefore, modern LMIC nursery building constructions are recommended to feature internal conduiting sleeves and inspection chambers that are specifically integrated for the installation of the PSS. The conduiting creates invaluable channels for the survival of many neonates who would soon require sharing the minimally available oxygen amongst themselves, simultaneously. The earlier version of the PSS was achieved via surface installation of its distribution sleeve round the internal perimeters of the nursery hall (**Figure 5**). However, fresh builds of nursery halls are equipped with predesigned internal conduit sleeves for this purpose.

6. Building with intent to mitigate neonatal infection and other deadly exposures

Neonatal infection has been implicated amongst the major causes of mortality in the newborn in Nigeria [14]. The efforts towards the prevention of a disease may always be cheaper than the huge and often unaffordable costs of treatment of infected patients. A variety of measures has been introduced as the standards of practice across Nigerian SCBUs, for example, to curb high neonatal infection rates. These include the use of 'sharps boxes', automatic electric hand driers that blow hot air, hand gloves and the use of hand sanitizing gels for the practitioners. Other measures include compulsory wearing of foot scrubs, gowns, and head covers for visitors at some Units. Observably, these sanitary measures are not equally enforced across all the SCBUs in Nigeria as most of these are completely missing in practices at so many facilities. These measures are considered helpful at other facilities; however, the practices are not strictly respected all the time, especially during the odd hours when high work pressure distracts the nurses from paying a full attention to the rules. Many of the managers agreed that enforcement of sanitary measures is also hampered by lack of specifically designated security officers to control visitor's traffic, as well as poor workflow due to the structural layout of the floor plan of their facility. The efficiency of these infection-curbing measures, where practiced, can improve or dwindle depending on the structural plan of the SCBU layout.

In our privileged inspection of over 50 SCBU facilities across more than 80% of the States of Nigeria, we can reveal that less than 10 of the SCBUs could be adjudged adequate to enable effective sanitary control. Habitually, the government and heads of hospitals in Nigeria do not seek sufficient professional consultations before the design and construction of hospitals. Adult patients in the adult facility wards may easily cope with most fallouts from poorly designed or constructed building. However, the relatively unknown protective features of a functional SCBU-building are often missing, hence, most of the Nigerian SCBU-buildings are lacking in the ability to better

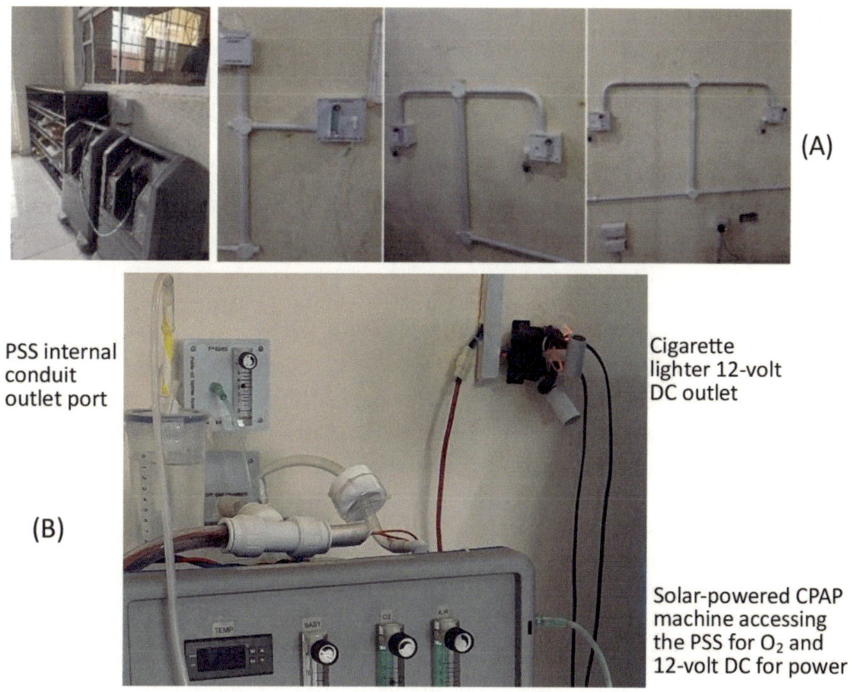

Figure 5.
The PSS (A) surface distribution sleeves (B) conduit installation.

protect the neonates. Unlike adult patients, the neonates are unable to cope, hence, some of them would die as a result. Therefore, it is essential that neonatal facilities are professionally earmarked and purposely structured during the design stage of any hospital facility. Purposeful and efficient neonatal building layout is one single factor amongst many considerations; however, it is one factor that saves huge amount of resources for LMIC practices when properly executed. Poor building positioning (as in defending against EFS) and structural layout (as in defending against infection) could be unquantifiably costly in losses of neonatal lives and in funding human traffic control, which could have been achieved naturally. Neonatal infection is caused by the propagation of bacteria that overpowers the non-immuned neonate. Infection could, therefore, be reduced by limiting the access of microbial vendors into the SCBU and by the application of a proper isolation-system for infected neonates. In this section, we highlight some often neglected aspects of SCBU positioning, layouts and features that could minimize infection and hence, neonatal deaths. Some of these features and specialized segments are usually difficult to adequately integrate into an already existing building through renovations, unless the building is substantially demolished to enable a better professional reconstruction. This is the concept our team applied in the newly reconstructed SCBU structure at the Federal Medical Centre, Owerri, Nigeria [15]. It is usually easier to conceptualize and integrate these into the original nursery building design ahead of construction.

Many channels of hospital infection are well-known adverse environmental conditions. Some of these adverse situations could be mitigated by a properly designed SCBU facility that specifically integrates important features as explained below:

1. **Exclusive neonatal transfer corridors linking the delivery and neonatal Units**. During facility accreditation for postgraduate training licensing, strict demands are made in Nigeria for SCBUs to be located very proximal to Labour Wards and obstetrics-theaters for aiding a quick and seamless transfer of newly-born neonates from the obstetrics to the neonatal wards. This, they argue, is essential for the protection of the fresh neonate from environmental pollutions during transfer, especially in the prevailing circumstance where most tertiary hospitals in Nigeria do not have functional transport incubators. Over the years, quite a few tertiary hospitals have been able to comply with this requirement through the modification of their centres, or re-allocating possible facility spaces to relocate the SCBU closer to the obstetrics units. However, some of these modifications have still failed to maximally isolate the transported neonate from the so-called environmental contagions as the newly born neonates still have to be moved through public-shared corridors to access the SCBU. It is evident that environmental pollution can be high at some LMIC settings, hence, a demand for an exclusive neonatal transfer corridor, which can naturally keep-off wandering members of the public and non-related hospital staff, remains as valid as all efforts to keep the neonates alive. Exclusive neonatal transfer corridors have been intentionally implemented in the modification of some recent Nigerian centres that were anchored by our research team, for example, the NRS hubcentres of Yobe State in northeast Nigeria (**Figure 6**).

2. **Specialized first-seven-days of life (F7D) room**. The higher vulnerability of neonates during their F7D period of life has been highlighted in the Nigerian demographic survey reports, showing that 4-of-5 deceased neonates would die at this stage [16]. This fact inspired the concept of the F7D room of our team.

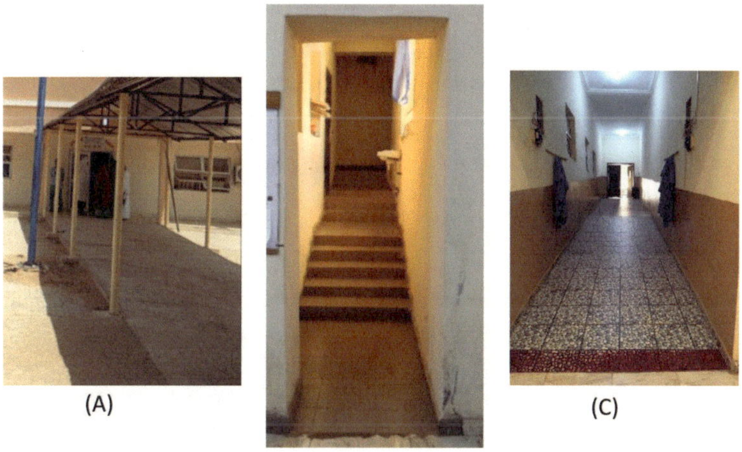

(A) (B) (C)

Figure 6.
Exclusive neonatal transfer corridor at Potiskum NRS hubcentre in Yobe State (A) public access to SCBU office sections (B) nursing mothers' exclusive access to milking/KMC rooms (c) neonate exclusive corridor linking Delivery room & SCBU.

Newly born neonates easily fall victims of cross-infection at Nigeria's busy SCBUs due to a habitual nursing staff shortage [8]. The ratio of on-duty nurses-to-neonates can easily get worse than 1:9, with neonates on admission ranging from the most vulnerable 'day-old extremely-low birthweight infants' to more tolerable 'full-term 20-days old' infants [13]. Feeding time and the associated extreme work pressure makes the overworked staff to attend to all neonates, moving continuously from one to another, often forgetting to observe the in-between washing of hands or change of gloves to avoid transmission of infection. Observably, our research team can affirm that this is habitual in the Nigerian practice, requiring only one nearly impossible solution, which is the employment of adequate staff strength. Cross-infection is a high-risk situation, especially to the few days' old more vulnerable preterm neonates who may not survive this. Inadequate staff strength can promote high cross-infection rate with its relatively higher consequences for the F7D-classified neonates. Staff employment is often a government policy, and uncontrollable by the local hospital management. However, an effective SCBU layout, which is controllable by the management, can help mitigate against cross-infection errors, which is common with inexperienced nurses. We created the F7D Room as an exclusive segment of the nursery hall where the premature and low birthweight neonates are nursed until their seventh day. The F7D nursing is only assigned to the best experienced nurses on duty rota.

3. **External Oxygen cylinder chambers instead of frequent cylinder traffics into the SCBU**. Most SCBUs across the regions of Nigeria do not operate on piped oxygen. Oxygen for daily work is supplied in oxygen-cylinders that are dragged right inside the SCBU, beside the cots and incubators, and maintained on refill-and-replace basis. Hence, the frequent back-&-forth movement of cylinders encourage transfer of microbes from dirty storage and gas-refilling shops via the indiscriminate entries of the 'dirty' gas technicians. Transmission of organisms owing to high traffic of dirty oxygen cylinders may be a major contributor to

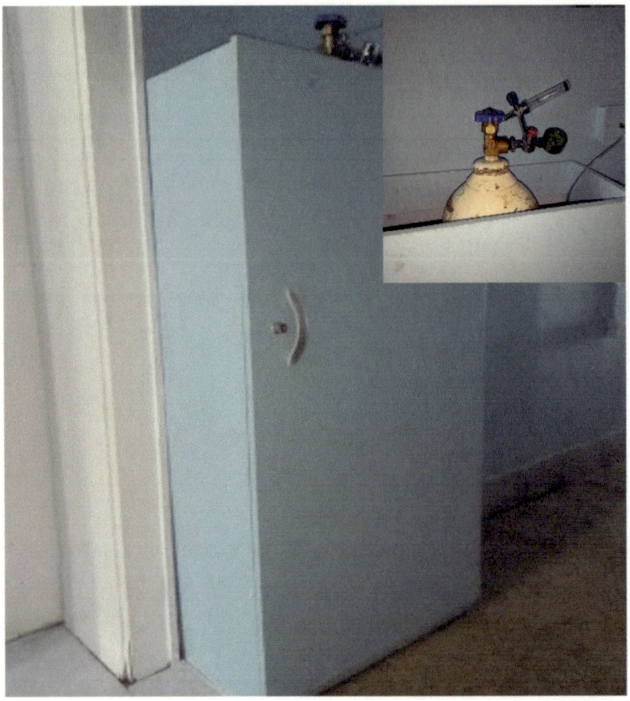

Figure 7.
External oxygen cylinder chambers behind the Neoroom walls at Calabar Women & Children Hospital (CWCH), Calabar, Nigeria.

high neonatal infection rate in Nigeria, and this needs to be studied. We proposed and implemented building designs with inbuilt oxygen cylinder chambers behind the walls of the SCBU and connected via short pipes across the walls into the SCBU's wall-mounted humidified flow gauges and controllers. Access to the cylinders is restricted with locks depending on how the chamber is exposed to passers-by (**Figure** 7).

4. **Mothers' dormitory exclusive access to the 'milking' and 'kangaroo mother care (KMC)' rooms**. Personal hygiene of nursing mothers is highly emphasized but may be easily implemented through some building enabled restrictions. Nurses, who are mostly women in Nigeria, assist in various inspections that help to educate and remind the mothers on the vital rules of hygiene to keep their babies safe. These needs inspired designs for adjoining mothers' dormitory with exclusive access to the milking and KMC rooms. The typical structure created by our team ensures private assistance of nurses to the nursing mothers through the exclusive corridor (**Figure 6B**). This allows mothers to enter the KMC room for any interaction with their own babies who are brought to them in the KMC room, without the mothers entering the main nursing nursery halls where the other neonates are.

The other building features include:

1. The integration of external public access to administrative and ward mangers' office without passing through the nursery's nursing halls by non-SCBU staff on duty.

2. The integration of access to the seminar and conference sections of the Unit without entering or passing through the nursery's nursing sections.

3. The integration of a scrub and gowning room and locating this just before the entrance of the nursery's nursing halls.

4. The integration and location of an independent 'septic or isolation' room for infectious neonates, with its exclusive cross-ventilation, separate from the rest of the nursery's nursing halls.

7. Building with intent to sustain high sanitary standards through running water supply

It is well-known, even at private homes, that availability of water is essential to keeping a good hygiene standards to reduce contaminations and diseases. The hospital environment is a setting too dangerous to compromise water availability due to high vulnerability of patients. It is difficult to operate an efficient hospital, even in the hinterlands of the LMICs, without adequate infection controls. Sanitary measures for minimisation of infection outbreaks are often mediated using sustainable running water supply through pipes and taps that are distributed around the facility. Lack of sustainable running water supply in hospitals at LMICs is widespread. This situation is easily observable in many well-known healthcare institutions in Nigeria, and as has been reported from other LMIC settings [17]. Although a situation of health practice without water may be horrifying to imagine from the standards at HICs, it is nevertheless, a situation that seems not to bother practitioners in these LMIC centres irrespective of the observable consequences of the spread of diseases and poor overall health outcomes.

Public infrastructure such as pipe borne water supply is either irregular or completely inexistent at many city settings in Nigeria where hospitals are located. Therefore, private borehole installation powered by electricity is the most common solution at these facilities. The drawback, however, remains the well-known epileptic public power supply to these centres and the high cost of fossil fuel to run power generators. Hence, the problem is a 'round the circle' nightmare. Needless to say that this is more terrible for facilities located in the hinterlands of the LMICs, where we must create a viable solution to support our NRS advocacy of "reversal of neonatal traffic by taking our medicine to the neonates where they are" to eliminate the transport-induced distress that worsens their death rates [4].

In our NRS facility designs, an appropriate segment of the building is featured with a stairway access to the loft or rooftop, where an appropriate flat surface is constructed for the installation of an overhead water tank that would be linked to supply the pipes and taps in the SCBU facility. Safety barriers are constructed to confine the tank against the wind and protect people accessing the tank platform from falling. A very simple pulley-crank-rope mechanism could be locally constructed on the provided barrier, with buckets tied to the two ends of the rope (**Figure 8**).

Water is delivered to the overhead tank via solar powered water pumps that lift water from the conventional underground tanks or locally dug wells, as normally seen in the rural areas. It is essential to apply low-cost sustainable techniques that the local people can manage to sustain without much external assistance. Therefore, the

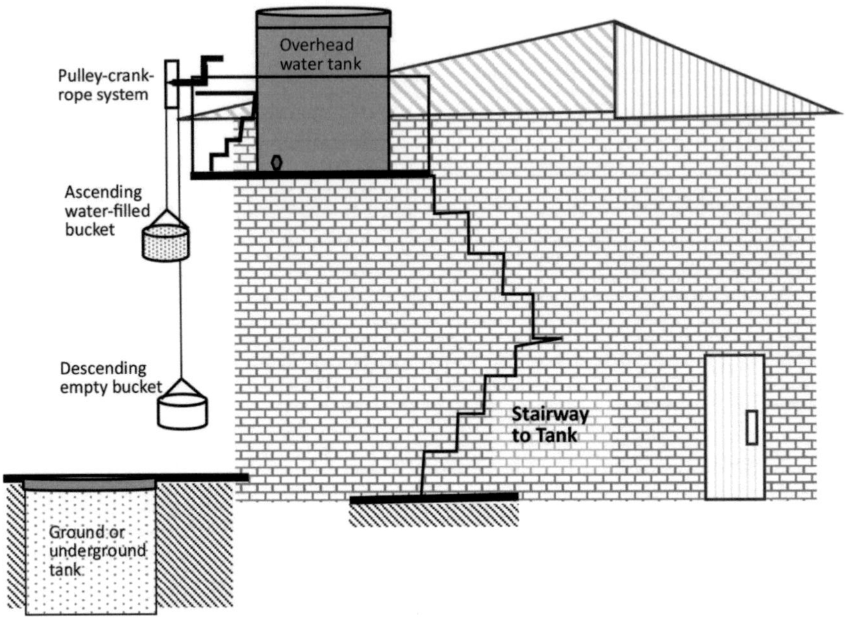

Figure 8.
Illustration of NRS-building featuring overhead water tank system.

low-voltage pumps, which are powered via our 12 VDC solar pannel gang (see Section 3), is the default method of lifting water into the overhead tank. At other likely times of pump failure, two other methods could be activated – manual and semi-manual. In the manual method, hospital oderlies would be required to climb the stair ways with water cans to fill up the overhead tank. The semi-manual option is performed by two persons, one on ground level refilling buckets and the other on the overhead tank platform, cranking the pulley-crank-rope system to lift water-filled bucket at one end of the rope whilst lowering an empty bucket for a re-fill at the other end of the rope (**Figure 8**). A servicing-hole with removable cork near the bottom of the overhead tank is used for a quick evacuation of contaminated water whenever this becomes necessary, or during the periodic washing of the tank. The orderlies are taught on how to use a 'provided' wash-stick for cleaning. The wash-stick is a construct of a long PVC pipe that is screwed to a spongy brush.

8. Final considerations

The nursery building is a vital equipment factor to consider without compromise in the setting up of a special care baby unit (SCBU) anywhere in the world. The LMICs are trailed with a lot of social and infrastructural limitations that often hinder the delivery of safe neonatal services, but little is known about possible building features and layouts that could effectively mitigate the effects of these limitations. Over the last 25 years, our group has carefully and consistently researched and implemented some of these various features, which are currently reaping good positive impacts.

A lot of SCBUs across Nigeria have benefitted from the wealth of knowledge so-generated through our research findings, trialing and implementations. In recent years, some freshly built or 'demolished-and-rebuilt' SCBUs have succeeded in the integration of a multitude of these individual features, simultaneously, thereby witnessing a delightful new experience of successful and safe neonatal environment. One of such efforts was implemented at Owerri, southeast of Nigeria. The re-engineering of the little space that accommodated what is referred to as the 'SCBU-1' of the Federal Medical Centre Owerri by our team in 2022, endaevoured to integrate as many of

S/N	Criteria (Score: 0–100%)		Details of criteria and scoring benchmarks	The Federal Medical Centre, Owerri	
1	Usage till date		How long has the new SCBU-1 been in use till date?	12 months	
2	Lighting coverage	The corridor	By how much satisfaction does the polite-light-bank (PLB) illumination sufficiently cover walking around safely at night without the need for extra lighting? No illumination (0%) – extremely sufficient (100%)	100 100 100 100 100	100%
		Inner SCBU		100 100 100 100 100	100%
3	Workflow		This relates to the nurse's sitting arrangement, ease of observation and swift attendance to the neonate on admission during nursing care [equal level as former (0%) – completely far better (100%)]	100 100 100 100 80	96%
4	Ease of reception of new patient		By what % improvement has the new building design made easier the process of admitting new neonates?	80 100 100 100 80	92%
5	Nurses' private areas		The new concepts of (1) napping couch and study privacy (2) storage and (3) showering. By how much % has this encouraged nursing efficiency and services	100 80 100 100 100	96%
6	Matron's office		The new concept created a kind of 'bird eyes' view for the matron from the comfort of her office desk. How does this compare to previous situations [gives her no better control (0%) – best effective control (100%)]	100 100 100 100 100	100%
7	Mini conference/ utility area		What is your fair score of this section?	100 100 100 100 80	96%
8	Mothers' milking cubicle		How do you score this privacy for milking mothers?	50 70 60 70 80	66%

S/N	Criteria (Score: 0–100%)	Details of criteria and scoring benchmarks	The Federal Medical Centre, Owerri	
9	Equipment base	How does the amount and caliber of installed equipment compare to your expectations? Poorer than expected (0%)..(100%) more than expected	80 80 80 100 100	88%
10	Overall satisfaction	What is your overall satisfaction rating for the ingenuity in this new concept compared to what you knew previously? No difference (0%)..maximally satisfied (100%)	100 80 90 100 100	94%

Five senior user nurses were discretely and unsuspectingly questioned by another colleague from a different hospital Unit specifically requesting: "if you scored the former "0%", how much could you score the new SCBU-1 on these criteria?"

Table 1.
Qualitative assessment of nursing functionality of the new SCBU-I compared to the former.

these features as possible. Thereby, a highly revolutionized practice setting was created. At the end of 12 months of continuous usage of the new SCBU-1, an interview team of two nurses from another department of the hospital was constituted. The team was commissioned to discretely target five unsuspecting senior nursing officers (SNO), who were longserving staff members of SCBU-1, to obtain their qualitative assessments of the new SCBU-1 as compared to the functionality of the demolished SCBU-1. The team applied a guided questionnaire technique involving a private informal chat session with the unsuspecting interviewee. It was necessary to apply this technique to avoid biased responses. Each of the five SNOs was interviewed separately by someone who was familiar, hence creating a friendly setting that encouraged the unsuspecting SNO to provide an honest comparison based on the content of the questionnaire (**Table 1**).

The obtained answers evidently show a strong agreement amongst the nurses that these features have made some remarkable impacts in their experiences. It is also noteworthy that all five interviewees expressed disappointment with the smallish capacity of the 'milking cubicle' as this could only take a maximum of five nursing mothers at a time. Therefore, each of the interviewees returned a low score for the cubicle. However, the question of size was a fundamental issue of the available land-space, which was too small to accommodate a larger room for the milking mothers.

Acknowledgements

We wish to thank our interviewers who helped us to achieve our unbiased assessment of the NRS-inspired designs of the special care baby units. This work was supported by Neonatal Concerns for Africa, a subsidiary of the Mastermind group, Nigeria. Professor Hippolite Amadi's outreach in Nigeria is supported by the Hornchurch Baptist Church, England, United Kingdom.

Conflict of interest

The authors declare no conflict of interest.

Author details

Hippolite O. Amadi[1*], Mohammed B. Kawuwa[2], Amina L. Abubakar[3] and Stephen K. Obaro[4]

1 Department of Bioengineering, Imperial College London, United Kingdom

2 Department of Obstetrics and Gynaecology, University of Maiduguri, Nigeria

3 Department of Obstetrics and Gynaecology, Kaduna State University, Nigeria

4 Section of Pediatrics Infectious Disease, University of Nebraska Medical Center, Omaha, USA

*Address all correspondence to: h.amadi@imperial.ac.uk

References

[1] Amadi HO, Adesina CT, Olateju EK, Omokaro S, Okechukwu AA, Alabi P, et al. Validation of a novel technique that minimises early neonatal deaths – A comparative study. Journal of Paediatrics and Neonatal Care. 2017;**6**(1):00232

[2] Amadi HO, Abubakar AL. LMIC facility-lighting limitation in Nigeria fully resolved by a novel frugal Polite-light-bank technology. Global Journal of Medical Research. 2023;**23**(3). Available from: https://globaljournals.org/GJMR_Volume23/1-LMIC-Facility-Lighting-Limitation-in-Nigeria.pdf

[3] Amadi HO. The Politeoxygen splitter system (PSS) – A frugal LMIC oxygen delivery technology that expands the utility by up to 700%. Journal of Paediatrics and Neonatal Care. 2023, 2023;**13**(2):75-80. DOI: 10.15406/jpnc.2023.13.00495. Available from: https://medcraveonline.com/JPNC/JPNC-13-00495.pdf

[4] Amadi HO, Kawuwa MB, Abubakar AL, Adesina CT, Olateju EK. A community integrated concept that minimises death of most vulnerable neonates at poor-resource environments. Journal of Paediatrics and Neonatal Care. 2022;**12**(3):170-173. DOI: 10.15406/jpnc.2022.12.00475

[5] Amadi HO, Mohammed IL, Kawuwa MB, Oyedokun A, Mohammed H. Synthesis and validation of a weather-proof nursery design that eliminates tropical Evening-Fever-Syndrome in neonates. International Journal of Paediatrics. 2014;**2014**:986760. DOI: 10.1155/2014/986760

[6] Amadi HO. Neonatal thermoneutrality in a tropical climate. In: Alfonso J. Rodriguez-Morales Ed, Current Topics in Tropical Medicine. London, UK: InTech Open, Croatia; 2012. p. 513-544. Available from: http://www.intechopen.com/books/current-topics-in-tropical-medicine/neonatal-thermoneutrality [Accessed March 16, 2012]

[7] Amadi HO, Olateju EK, Kawuwa MB, Osibogun AO, Alabi P, Ibadin MO. Neonatal hyperthermia and thermal stress in low- and middle-income countries: A hidden cause of death in extremely low-birthweight neonates. Paediatrics and International Child Health. 2015;**35**(3):273-281. Available from: http://www.maneyonline.com/doi/pdfplus/10.1179/2046905515Y.0000000030

[8] Uchendu C, Windle R, Blake H. Perceived facilitators and barriers to Nigerian Nurses' engagement in health promoting behaviors: A socio-ecological model approach. International Journal of Environmental Research and Public Health. 2020;**17**(4):1314. DOI: 10.3390/ijerph17041314

[9] Adair-Rohani H, Zukor K, Bonjour S, Wilburn S, Kuesel AC, Hebert R, et al. Limited electricity access in health facilities of sub-Saharan Africa: A systematic review of data on electricity access, sources, and reliability. Global Health Science Practise. 2013;**1**(2):249-261. DOI: 10.9745/GHSP-D-13-00037

[10] Ohajianya AC, Abumere OE, Owate IO, Osarolube E. Erratic power supply in Nigeria: Causes and solutions. International Journal of Engineering Science Invention. 2014;**3**(7):51-55

[11] Ekanem EE, Fajola AO, Ogbimi R, OgievaB JI. Use of solar energy for the provision of cost-effective and environmentally friendly power supply

in health facilities in the developing world- lessons from a community cottage hospital in Southern Nigeria. International Journal of Research Science & Management. 2014;**4**(4):32-37. DOI: 10.5281/zenodo.546865

[12] Amadi HO, Kawuwa MB. 2018. Reducing early neonatal mortality in Nigeria – the solution. Selected Topics in Neonatal Care. Barria R Mauricio. London, UKInTech Open, Croatia, 221-237 10.5772/intechopen.69221. https://www.intechopen.com/books/selected-topics-in-neonatal-care/reducing-early-neonatal-mortality-in-nigeria-the-solution [Accessed November 13, 2018]

[13] Amadi HO, Osibogun AO, Eyinade O, Kawuwa MB, Uwakwem AC, Ibekwe MU, et al. Challenges and frugal remedies for lowering facility based neonatal mortality – A comparative study. International Journal of Paediatrics. 2014;**2014**:986716. DOI: 10.1155/2014/986716

[14] Odejimi A, Quinley J, Eluwa GI, Kunnuji M, Wammanda RD, Weiss W, et al. Causes of deaths in neonates and children aged 1-59 months in Nigeria: Verbal autopsy findings of 2019 Verbal and Social Autopsy study. BMC Public Health. 2022;**22**(1):1130. DOI: 10.1186/s12889-022-13507-z

[15] Neonatal Concerns for Africa. A Range of Solar Powered Devices that Enables Neonatal Intervention at Remote Locations – FMC Owerri Video Report. 2022. https://www.youtube.com/watch?v=lAC0H-CwOSc [Accessed June 2, 2023]

[16] MCA, World Health Organisation. Maternal and Perinatal Health Profile of Nigeria, Africa Region. Maternal and Perinatal Country Profile [Internet]. Available from: http://www.who.int/maternal_child_adolescent/epidemiology/profiles/maternal/nga.pdf [Accessed: February 02, 2017]

[17] Chawla SS, Gupta S, Onchiri FM, Habermann EB, Kushner AL, Stewart BT. Water availability at hospitals in low- and middle-income countries: Implications for improving access to safe surgical care. Journal of Surgical Research. 2016;**205**:169-178. DOI: 10.1016/j.jss.2016.06.040

Chapter 3

Warmth, Food and Security – Triad of Neonatal Care and Safety

Tridibesh Tripathy, Shankar Das, Dharmendra Pratap Singh, Sovesh Chandra Tripathy, Anjali Tripathy, Sanskriti Tripathy, Rakesh Dwivedi and Mohini Gautam

Abstract

This chapter deals with the first month of life of the newborns in India. Although it is a global issue, the chapter focuses on the issue giving the history, perspective, current situation, and the future of newborns in India. Being the second most populous country in the world, the lessons learnt from India on neonatal care can be adopted by other countries. The application of the neonatal care on a large scale in India has been slow and gradual as it needs a multidimensional strategy. The neonatal care is at two poles. One at the in-reach and the other at the level of out-reach. The former is at the institutional level and the later at the institutional level. Both the concepts are detailed out in the chapter. The chapter also factors in the multiheaded dependent indicator, such as neonatal mortality rate, that impacts poverty, and thus social development. The chapter discusses the child survival interventions through the reduction of child mortality in India and aspires that India achieve the sustainable development goal related to child mortality.

Keywords: home-based newborn care, facility-based newborn care, Kangaroo Mother Care, colostrum, sample registration system, neonatal mortality rate, infant mortality rate, under five mortality rate

1. Introduction

As per the Hindu religious scripture, the Bhagwat Gita, Lord Krishna, a prominent Hindu god had an extremely turbulent life during his neonatal days [1]. The same struggle continues for all the current newborns or the birth cohort in India even today. The current neonatal mortality rate in India is 20 per 1000 live births as per SRS, 2020, and 24.9 as per NFHS 5 [2, 3]. The high neonatal mortality is primarily through the early neonatal mortality rate (ENMR) that occurs in the first week of life. The current ENMR is 15 per 1000 live births. The late neonatal mortality rate that occurs in the rest 3 weeks is 5 per 1000 live births. This chapter focuses on aspects toward reducing this mortality rate. India has two approaches to reduce neonatal mortality, which is on the lines of the World Health Organization's guidelines. These two approaches are home-based neonatal care (HBNC) practices and the facility-based neonatal care (FBNC) practices. The chapter focuses firstly on the HBNC approach [4].

Secondary data is the mainstay of the chapter. The chapter explores the gap between the current essential newborn care (EBNC) practices and HBNC practices. Through the gap exploration, the chapter finds out if there is a functional link between the two care approaches. Finally, the chapter suggests steps to be taken in future [4].

The current National Health Policy of India is viable till 2025, that is, 5 years before the SDG deadline. Therefore, it is envisaged that in next 2 years from now, the detail plans to introduce new and effective concepts in EBNC will be developed. The chapter also aspire that all the critical stakeholders of the sub national and national level will be involved to develop such detail plans. This will be a progressive step to fulfill the intricacies of the developed plan. Thereafter, India will be in a position to achieve the sustainable development goals (SDG) by 2030 and particularly those goals that are made toward reduction of neonatal, infant, and child mortality [5].

There are two aspects in the chapter. One is the community setting and the other is the hospital setting. The home-based newborn care (HBNC) is toward the community setting and the facility-based newborn care (FBNC) addresses the hospital setting. A child with a birth weight of less than 1800 grams has to be in the institutional care, whereas a child with birth weight more than 1800 grams can be saved through HBNC approaches [6].

The chapter is intended for people who are passionate about mother and child health (MCH). Among MCH, the chapter deals with the first month of life. It combines both the home-based newborn care (HBNC) and facility-based newborn care (FBNC) strategies in the most and densely populous country of the world, India. It deciphers out all the activities that can be done at home and facility levels to save the lives of all newborns. The chapter deals with the saving life or the need triad, especially for newborns. The three components of the triad are food, warmth, and security [6].

As all the HBNC-related activities are to be done at the grassroot level, the current chapter mentions the indicators through the work of the large network of outreach workers. These outreach workers are the Accredited Social Health Activists (ASHA) in India. These are daughters-in-law of the villages who work as volunteers. They are appointed by the local self-governance (LSG) to work on health-related issues in their own villages. They are attached to the public health system (PHS) by the LSGs. The PHS pays them honorariums for the various health services that they do at the grassroot level [6, 7].

As per the data of the Ministry of Health & Family Welfare (MOHFW) of Government of India, currently, there are 1 million ASHAs in India. They are spread over 18 Empowered Action Group (EAG) states or subnational levels. The National Health Mission was launched in 2005 in India in these 18 EAG states. As part of neonatal care package in India, home-based newborn care (HBNC) is one of the primary tasks of ASHAs. They are scheduled to visit homes of newborns to give need specific and time-based counseling at home level. Following such home visits, ASHAs are also supposed to refer the sick newborns, thus contributing to facility-based newborn care (FBNC) approaches. Among all the states in India, the most populous state in Northern India, the state of Uttar Pradesh has 0.15 million ASHAs from among the total 1 million in India [6, 7].

Subsequently, the chapter explores the history of newborn care in India and reaches to the current situation of the two elements of neonatal care, which are FBNC and HBNC. A comparison is done among the two elements in terms of modalities such as services, roll out and indicators of achievements through large-scale health surveys in India. These surveys include critical indicators on newborn care. Through this process, the importance of the triad of neonatal care, which is "warmth,", "food," and "security" in both the elements/approaches of newborn care are discussed. It is significant to note that the approach and criteria used to assess these two elements through the neonatal triad vary significantly [6–8].

The institutional care includes newborns whose birth weight is less than or equal to 1.8 kilograms as these kids should be under the purview of institutional care as per the prescribed guidelines of the Government of India (GoI). The guidelines are developed as per the World Health Organization guidelines on neonatal care. Under institutional care, besides the birth weight criteria, the sick newborns are also included in the FBNC approach. The institutional care has a three-tier approach in the public health system (PHS) in India. The first tier is the urban or rural primary health centers (UPHC/RPHC) that covers 30,000 to 40,000 population on an average. Here, the newborn care corners (NBCC) are established. Next tier is the community health center (CHC) that covers 0.1 million population on an average. In this tier, the newborn stabilization unit (NBSU) is set up. In the topmost tier, the new born care unit (NBCU) is established at the district-level hospitals or other health units, such as first referral units (FRU) that cover about 1.5 million populations. So, it is seen that the first two tiers operate at the sub-district level and the topmost tier is at the district level [6, 8].

The highest neonatal therapeutic unit is the medical college hospitals or the research institutions/higher medical centers that have neonatal intensive care units (NICU). These cater to the cases such as defects at birth or sick and premature babies that are born during the viability period of 180 to 210 days. These newborns need special care that is given by staffs trained on neonatal care. The current annual birth cohort of India is 250 million. Hence, the newborn care becomes critical as it is the ladder to reduce not only neonatal mortality rate (NMR) but also the infant mortality rate (IMR) and the under 5 mortality rate (U5MR) as well finally impacting the overall child mortality (CM). This is how it addresses the human development index (HDI) and other social development indicators (SDI) of the country. Further, it is seen that the all-important multidimensional poverty index (MDPI) used internationally also focuses on the child mortality rate (CMR) as a crucial indicator. Hence, it is a fact that any road to reduction in CMR has to navigate through a reduction in NMR and especially the ENMR [8–11].

2. History of newborn care in India

The historical perspective of FBNC and HBNC programs in India needs to be understood to comprehend the current situation of India in terms of neonatal care. The following box shows this historical progress through a time line. In short, it is the mirror of neonatal care of India (**Box 1**) [6–11].

This chapter focuses on both the FBNC and HBNC, which are part of child health intervention (CHI) in India. It is imperative to trace the history of the child survival programs in India as the neonatal care is its base. In the beginning, the focus of child survival intervention was on the operation of immunization programs in India. In India in 1978 through the expanded program on immunization (EPI), the child survival interventions saw the light of the day. The section below has the details related to the entire gamut of development of newborn care in India [12].

A district newborn care program was initiated as part of CSSM in 26 selected districts in India almost 30 years ago in 1994. It led to the development of the national

Box 1

- 1980—National neonatology forum (NNF) launched. The next step was taken after 12 years.
- 1992—Essential newborn care (ENC) launched through Child Survival and Safe Motherhood (CSSM) program. First time, maternal and child health was seen as a single component.
- 1994—In 26 districts of India, newborn care program (NCP) launched through CSSM. First time, experiments or interventions were done at subnational level.
- 1994—National program on facility-based newborn care (FBNC) launched. Subsequent to the subnational efforts, the national-level effort was initiated.
- 2000—National Newborn Week (NNW) initiated and to be celebrated from fifteenth to twenty-first November each year. A dedicated time was ascribed to the newborn care on the lines of WHO.
- 2003—District-level newborn care unit (NBU) set up in Purulia district, West Bengal. The FBNC effort was demonstrated successfully at the subnational level.
- 2011—Home-based newborn care (HBNC) guidelines launched. The newborn care moved from the facility level to the community level.
- 2013—Integrated action plan for prevention and control of pneumonia and diarrhea (IAPPD) launched. This framework was developed subsequent to the integrated management of neonatal and childhood illnesses (IMNCI) framework. The community level framework was C-IMNCI, and the facility level framework was F-IMNCI.
- 2013—RMNCH+A launched in the month of February. First time, the focus shifted to adolescents and reproductive Health. The framework provides the care and services to be provided in a 5*5 framework.
- 2014—India Newborn Action Plan launched. This comprehensive document combines both the FBNC and HBNC strategies.
- 2015—Neonatal mortality rate became the first step toward reduction of infant mortality rate. India adopted the launch of goal #3 of sustainable development goals (SDG) by United Nations. At the national level, alignment of the national strategy was done with the SDG since 2015. This was followed after the roll out of millennium development goals (MDG) that was operational during the 2000–2015 period.

program on FBNC in the same year. The percolation of these efforts led to creations of newborn care corners (NBCC) at every point of childbirth across the nation. Subsequent to that, newborn stabilization units (NBSU) at First Referral Units (FRU) and Special Newborn Care Units (SNCU) at district hospitals came up [13].

Almost after 10 years of this event, in the year 2003, in Purulia district of the state of West Bengal in India, for the first time, it was demonstrated that institutional-level care of newborns is feasible at the district level. A triad level of care is detailed out in the FBNC guidelines of GOI. The first level is care at birth, the second level is care of normal newborn, and the third level is the care of sick newborn. The national-level experience of 11 years on newborn care led to the development of India Newborn Action Plan (INAP) in the year 2014. This GOI document details out the Standard Operating Procedures (SOP) of both the HBNC and FBNC components [8, 9, 12–17].

3. HBNC vs. FBNC

As mentioned above, a child has to have a birth weight of at least 1800 grams to qualify for HBNC or stay at home. The HBNC approach is meaningless without the need and support of outreach health providers. Only places where the outreach worker visits the homes of pregnant women in their last trimester of pregnancy, those places can only ensure the benefit of the triad of warmth, food, and security [4, 6].

This paragraph details out the activities that need to be done to maintain the warmth of the child. The first activity is drying and wrapping the child immediately after birth. The second activity is to give skin-to-skin contact (STSC) by the mothers or any other caregiver. Here, the child gets the warmth of the mother or caregiver through the skin of the mother or caregiver. The point of caution is that the mother or caregiver should not have any cloth between the newborn and herself or himself. Both the child and the mother and caregiver should be covered from the top. The newborn should be kept in frog position between the breasts of the mother or caregiver with the mouth and nose sideways so that the child can respire or breathe freely. Humans learned the technique from the Kangaroos. The newborn of the Kangaroo lies in the pouch of the mother Kangaroo. The newborn derives warmth from the skin of the mother Kangaroo's pouch. The newborn of the Kangaroo breastfeeds himself or herself while within the pouch [6–8].

This is how the newborn of the human or Kangaroo safely travels the first 28 days of life. It is rightly said and proved that the mother or the caregiver is the best warmer for the child leave aside the Radiant Warmer (RW) that are put up in institutions for neonatal care [8, 18].

The third activity to maintain warmth is through the delay of the bathing of the newborn at least for the ENMR period so that the Vernix Caseosa or the natural blanket that the newborn has on his or her skin is not removed. The ENMR period is for the first week of life. This process ensures that hypothermia in the newborn is prevented and taken care of [18].

The second component is the food component of newborn. The food component is attributed to the exclusive breastfeeding (EBF) practices of the child. The EBF period is during the 0–6 months of life. The EBF practice stipulates that only three things are allowed orally for the child in the first 6 months of life. These are oral rehydration solution (ORS) in case of neonatal diarrhea. The second thing is the oral vaccines (Polio and Rota), and the third thing is the prescribed medicines in case of a sickness in the newborn. The newborn should not be given anything orally till he or she attains 6 months of age other than these three things that are allowable orally. Water is also not allowed as the breast milk of the lactating mother has enough water for the child. The foremilk in both the breasts of the mother quenches the thirst of the newborn. Similarly, the hind milk in both the breasts of the mothers satiates the hunger of the newborn. So, the newborn drinks first and eats next unlike the adults [8, 18].

The third component addresses the security aspect of the child. Here, the activity is that the newborn should not be left alone in any case during the first month of life. The mother and the caregivers should be vigil and secure the newborn 24*7 [8, 18].

The KMC package bifurcates into STSC- and EBF-related activities. All the activities mentioned above can be done at household or home without any intervention or support from the skilled staff of the entire health system. That is why the package is called as HBNC package. In the first month of life that is highly sensitive, it should be ensured that there should not be a moving fan and no working air conditioner in the newborn's room. All these activities further add to more loss of heat from the body of the newborn. The windows of the room are to be kept open to help the mother, caregiver, and the newborn to breathe freely. Every day as a routine, the newborn needs exposure to the morning sun for 15 minutes on an average. All such activities at home and institution lead to keeping the newborn warm, thus reducing the chances of mortality from hypothermia [6, 8, 18].

Next in line is the food component that addresses the indicators, such as early initiation of breastfeeding (EIBF) or Colostrum Feeding (CF). The former indicator holds good in the first 3 days of life, and the latter indicator holds good for the rest 27 days of life [8, 17].

4. Newborn care-related indicators in large-scale surveys in India

One of the large-scale surveys in India that captures newborn-related data is the National Family Health Survey (NFHS) that started in 1992–1993. It is done by the Ministry of Health & Family Welfare (MoHFW) of the Government of India (GOI), where the coordinating institution is the International Institute of Population Sciences located in Mumbai in the state of Maharashtra in India. It is an autonomous institution under the MoHFW of the GOI. Till the year 2023, there have been five rounds of this survey in India. **Table 1** shows the newborn care-related indicators and their performance through the five rounds of these NFHS surveys [2, 3].

Survey Rounds & Year of survey	Newborn care-related indicators	Performance of the indicators in percentage
NFHS-I, 1992–1993	1. Children 0–1 month who are breastfeeding 2. Children under 3 years of age breastfed within 1 hour of birth	1. 97.8 2. 9.5
NFHS-2, 1998–1999	1. Children 0–3 months exclusively breastfed 2. Median duration of breast feeding in months 3. Children under 3 years of age breastfed within 1 hour of birth	1. 55.2 2. 25.4 3. 16.0
NFHS-3, 2005–2006	1. Children under 3 years of age breastfed within 1 hour of birth 2. Children 0–5 months exclusively breastfed 3. Children born at home who were taken to a health facility for checkup within 24 hours of birth	1. 23.4 2. 46.4 3. 0.3
NFHS-4, 2015–2016	1. Children born at home who were taken to a health facility for checkup within 24 hours of birth 2. Children who received a health check after birth from a doctor/nurse/LHV/ANM/Midwife/other health personnel within 2 days of birth 3. Children under 3 years of age breastfed within 1 hour of birth 4. Children under 6 months of age exclusively breastfed	1. 2.5 2. 27.2 3. 41.6 4. 54.9
NFHS-5, 2019–2021	1. Neonatal mortality rate 2. Children under 3 years breastfed within 1 hour of birth 3. Children under 6 months of age exclusively breastfed	1. 24.9 (Per 1000 Live births). This number is an absolute number and not in percentage. 2. 41.8 3. 63.7

Table 1.
Newborn care-related indicators in NFHS [2].

The other sources of data related to newborns, which are live births, stillbirths, and neonatal mortality, are given by the sample registration system (SRS) in India. The SRS was piloted in 1964–1965, and the system became fully operational in 1969–1970. Prior to SRS, the civil registration system (CRS) that included registration of births and deaths was operational on a voluntary basis after independence in 1947. The CRS was not uniform statistically as there were cases of under-registration and suboptimal coverage. In order to streamline the CRS-related activities, the registration of Births & Deaths Act, 1969 was enacted by the Indian parliament. To further strengthen and streamline the statistical data in India, the SRS was started as an alternative to the CRS. Currently, both the CRS and SRS co-exist [3, 9–11].

The following figures show SRS data related to child mortality, where it can be inferred that reduction in neonatal mortality rate (NMR) will eventually lead to reduction in infant mortality rate (IMR) and under 5 mortality rate (U5 MR). A slow reduction of NMR has led to slow reduction in both IMR and U5MR [3].

From the three figures, it can be seen that from 2014 to 2020, only a six-point reduction in NMR led to an 11-point reduction in IMR and 13-point reduction in U5 MR. This means a point reduction in NMR leads to almost two-point reduction in IMR and slightly more than double reduction in U5 MR. The inferred reduction ratio formula in the child mortality rates in India from 2014 to 2020 is NMR: IMR: U5MR is 6:11:13 or 1:1.8; 2.1 [3].

This is where the approach of FBNC and HBNC is critical as these approaches reduce the early neonatal mortality rate (ENMR), which takes into account the deaths in first week of life or in the 0–6 days of life. The period from 7 to 28 days falls under late neonatal mortality rate (LNMR). Currently, in India, the NMR is 20 per 1000 live births, the ENMR is 15 per 1000 live births, and the LNMR is 5 per 1000 live births. Hence, the complete focus should be on the first 7 days of life so that 15/20*100 = 75% of neonatal deaths are prevented. It is here that the neonatal triad along with the proven child survival interventions, such as immunizations, has a big role to play in reduction of NMR in India. The concept of deaths of newborns in India in the first 7 days of life has been discussed in the chapter in another section. Similarly, the current immunization for newborn is also discussed in the chapter in another section given below (**Figures 1–3**) [3].

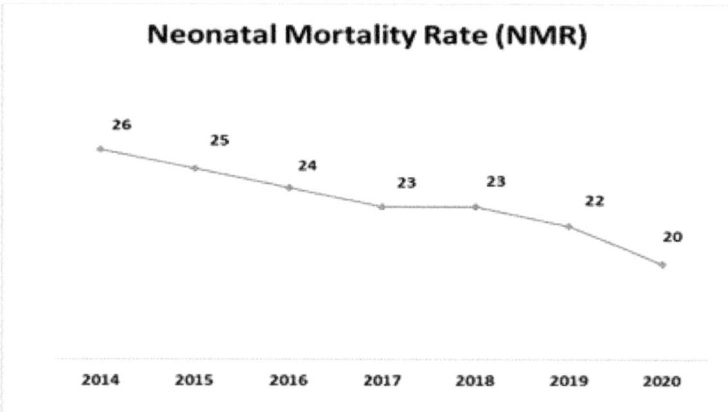

Figure 1.
NMR in India [3]—Chart by the lead author.

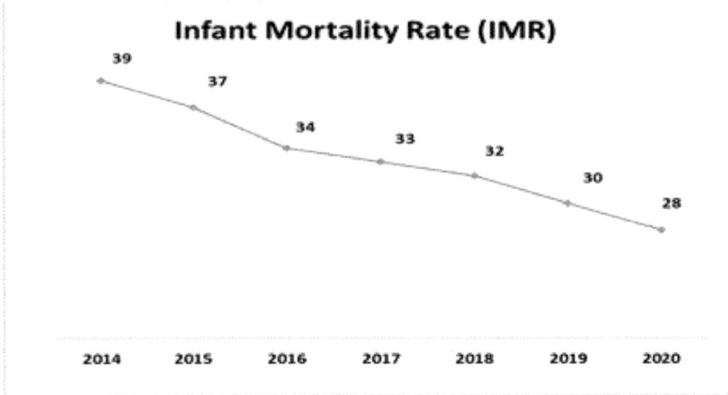

Figure 2.
IMR in India (source-SRS, 2020)[3]—Chart by the lead author.

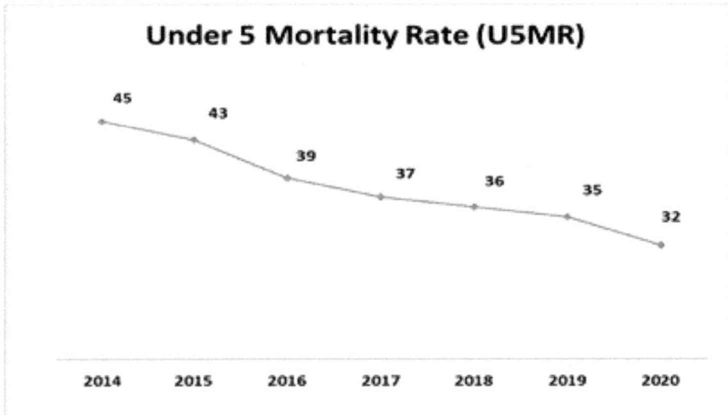

Figure 3.
U5 MR in India (SRS, 2020) [3]—Chart by the lead author.

5. Current immunization schedule in India

In India, currently, the campaign regarding immunization is "5 years, 7 times and not to drop a single time." This means till 5 years of age, the child has to attend the vaccination centers seven times, where the vaccinator will vaccinate the child as per prescribed immunization schedule. **Table 2** gives the details of the current immunization schedule in India. The current article focuses on the immunization of newborns that addresses the prevention aspects of newborns [12].

As seen from the above table, at birth, the child is vaccinated with BCG to prevent from tuberculosis, hepatitis B to prevent from serum hepatitis, and the zero dose for prevention from poliomyelitis. With this, the neonatal stage of the vaccination schedule finishes for the child. Hence, it is inferred that the newborn is prevented from tuberculosis, serum hepatitis, and poliomyelitis through three different vaccinations in the first month of life [12, 14, 17].

Age of the child in months/ years	Prescribed vaccinations
At birth (first time)	Bacillus Calmette Guerrin (BCG), Hepatitis B, Polio (Zero Dose)
At one and half months (second time)	Pentavalent-1, OPV-1, fipv-1, Rota-1, PCV-1
At two and half months (third time)	Pentavalent-2, OPV-2, Rota-2
At three and half months (fourth time)	Pentavalent-3, OPV-3, fipv-2, Rota-3, PCV-2
At 9–12 months (fifth time)	MR-1, JE-1, PCV-B, fipv-3, vitamin-A-1
At 16–24 months (sixth time)	MR-B, JE-B, DPT-1, vitamin-A-2nd to 6th dose at every 6-month interval
At 5–6 years (seventh time)	DPT-2
For Pregnant Women	Td-1 and Td-2 at an interval of 3 months between the two doses. Td-B one dose given to the mother if there is a gap of less than 3 years between two pregnancies.

Pentavalent stands for a combination of five vaccines such as Diphtheria, Pertussis, Tetanus, Hepatitis B, and Haemophilus Influenzae type B (Hib).
OPV stands for Oral Polio Vaccine.
The acronym "fipv" stands for fractional inactivated polio vaccine.
Rota vaccine is given for diarrhea.
PCV stands for Pneumococcal Conjugate Vaccine.
MR stands for Measles & Rubella.
JE stands for Japanese Encephalitis that is given to children in selected states of Uttar Pradesh, Andhra Pradesh, Bihar, and Telangana.
DPT stands for Diphtheria, Pertussis and Tetanus.
Td stands for Tetanus and a small diphtheria component.
B stands for booster dose.

Table 2.
Routine immunization schedule of India, 2023 [12, 14].

6. PPT of newborns

The protection, prevention, and treatment (PPT) model is adopted to deal with neonatal care. The following table details out the model. It is to be noted that protection component comes only once in a lifetime for the newborn. These are the Early Initiation of Breast Feeding (EIBF), which is commonly known as colostrum feeding that lasts for only 3 days after birth followed by the exclusive breast feeding (EBF) that lasts for 4–28 days for the newborn. This is the "food" component of the newborn [17].

Besides immunization, the other prevention-related activities of the newborn are drying, wiping, and wrapping the newborn after birth so that the warmth is maintained. The other activities, such as not bathing the newborn for 7 days, providing Skin to Skin Care (STSC) as a part of the Kangaroo Mother Care (KMC), not using air conditioner or fans in the newborn's room and showing the morning sun to the newborn for 15 minutes also maintains the warmth of the baby. These activities are preventive activities for the newborn to prevent him/her from hypothermia [18].

Keeping a constant vigil on the newborn addresses the security component of the newborn triad. This is also a preventive activity for the newborn [8].

Protection	Prevention	Treatment
• The first protective activity is "Colostrum Feeding" which is technically known as Initiation of Breast Feeding that should be given ideally within 1 hour of birth. • The second protective activity is Exclusive Breastfeeding that should be done from 0 to 6 months of age for every child. The orally allowed substances for the newborn during this period are oral vaccines such as Polio & Rota, Oral Rehydration Solution (ORS) if the newborn suffers from diarrhea or dehydration and prescribed medicines if the newborn falls sick.	• Hand washing with soap before 7 critical action points. These are before preparing food for the child, after cleaning the child's toilet, after household chores, before eating, before serving food and before feeding the child. • Clean and potable drinking water for the mother, child, and clean air to breathe in both indoor &and outdoor. • Use of functional and clean toilets by all the household members, masks for members of the household having respiratory issues, vaccines such as OPV-Zero dose, Hepatitis B and BCG, • Therapeutic measures such as Cotrimoxazole prophylaxis for HIV infected and exposed newborns	• Improved & timely care seeking & referral of sick newborns. • Case management of sick newborns at health facility/ institutions & community/ grassroot level • Cotrimoxazole for not severe Acute Respiratory Infection (ARI) cases, amoxicillin for severe ARI cases • Oxygen for ARI in newborn in health facilities • ORS but no Zinc supplement for newborn having diarrhea as Zinc is not given to 0–2-month-old child. • Continued feeding including breastfeeding for Young Children & only EBF for newborns.

Table 3.
PPT model as per IAPPD [17].

In case of any danger signs in the newborn, the newborn should be referred for treatment to a center, where sick newborn care unit exists or to a higher level of health care, where neonatal intensive care unit is functional. This addresses the treatment part of the newborn. **Table 3** relates to the PPT framework [8].

The table has mentions of diarrhea and pneumonia as these are the two major killers of newborns [19].

7. Major killers of newborns at global level

The following section deals with the major killers of children under 5 years of age, where the neonatal deaths contribute to 57.9% of all deaths and the rest is for the postnatal stage. Among the three diseases, such as tetanus, diarrhea, and pneumonia, there are two major killers, which continue in the postnatal period as well. These two are diarrhea and pneumonia that are a threat for children till 5 years of age. That leaves us only with tetanus that is a potential threat to the newborn. Among newborns, diarrhea contributes to 0.4% of all deaths and pneumonia contributes to 3%. The rest all are conditions that are a danger to the newborn. The contexts of these two major killers are mentioned in the above PPT framework through the mention of treatment of pneumonia and diarrhea. The causes of U5 deaths in global level apply to India, as well as these cohort studies are done on a large scale and over a period of time [17, 19].

8. Neonatal mortality and multidimensional poverty index (MPI)

The global MPI includes education, health, and standard of living as the three dimensions to measure poverty. Unlike the previous methods that included income and consumption as the indicators. In the MPI, there are three dimensions and 10 indicators. Each of the dimensions has one-third weightage. The details of the dimension and the related indicators are given below as per the weightage [10].

The first is the education dimension. Under this dimension, there are two indicators. These are "Years of Schooling" and "Child Enrollment." Each of these indicators has 1/6 weightage. When we sum up 1/6 + 1/6, we get 1/3 [10].

The second is the health dimension. The indicators under this dimension are "child mortality" and "nutrition." Each of the two indicators has 1/6 weightage. Thus, on adding them, we get 2/6 or 1/3 [10].

Under the third dimension comes the standard of living. In this dimension, there are six indicators. These indicators are "electricity," "flooring," "drinking water," "sanitation," "cooking Fuel," and "assets." Each of these indicators has 1/18 weightage. On adding the weightage of each of these indicators, we get 6/18 or 1/3 [10].

Hence, each dimension through their related indicators contributes to one third of the poverty measure scale. The total poverty is represented as 1 adding 1/3 + 1/3 + 1/3 = 3/3 = 1 [10].

The index cites that a person/household will be categorized as multi-dimensionally poor when deprived in one third or more or 33% or more of the weighted all the 10 indicators of the three dimensions [10].

In case, the deprivation is half or more of the weighted indicators, these households are clubbed under extreme multidimensional poverty. It should be noted that the MPI ranges from "0" to "1," where higher values mean higher level of poverty [10].

Here, we can see that one third of the weightage revolves around child mortality. The poor households need support from the public health system through the outreach and in-reach platforms so that they can save their newborns, which, in turn, will help reduce infant mortality and finally impact U5 mortality. Through reduction in these three stages of neonant, infant, and U5, we can reduce child mortality. Hence, poverty is rightly seen as a state of health in epidemiology and child mortality as an indicator of social development [9–11, 14].

9. Growth and development in newborn

The term "growth" means increase in the physical size of the body that we measure in terms of system international (SI) units, such as kilograms and centimeters. "Development" means increase in skill and function. These two are termed together as the child grows and develops as a whole. These two terms not only talk about physical aspects but also include intellectual, emotional, and social aspects of newborns. Data related to growth and development includes a comprehensive and sensitive indicator specific to child health that starts with the newborn health before and after birth [20, 21].

The growth chart tracks the growth and development through weight as the numerator and age as the denominator. Here, weight is the dependent variable, and age is the independent variable. A newborn usually doubles its birth weight by 5 months and trebles it by the end of the first year. For example, a newborn with 2.5

kilograms at birth will be 5 kilograms by 5 months of age, thus gaining 500 grams per month. Among these 5 months, the first month is the most critical as the newborn has to gain 500 grams by the end of neonatal stage. This is only possible if the triad of warmth, food, and security are adhered with as per standards [20, 21].

Similarly, the height/length of newborn is 50 cm, and it should be 75 cm by the end of the first year of life. So every month, the newborn is expected to gain 2 cm. Here again, the gain of 2 cm in the first month is most critical. If these two indicators are taken care of, the crossing over of chest and head circumferences takes place in the infancy stage. All these growths and development-related indicators are achievable only if the food component of the newborn is taken care of. The following section deals with the care protocol component of newborns [20–22].

10. Care protocol for babies in India

Government of India's Ministry of Health & Family Welfare developed a document titled "National Patient Safety Implementation framework for the period of 2018–2025 aligning the document with the end line of the current National Health Policy (NHP)." The patient safety is a fundamental element of public health care. The document defines the concept "as the freedom for a patient from unnecessary harm or potential harm associated with provision of health care" [23].

For the safety of the newborns, there are provisions and checks against issues such as inadvertent mix-up of babies at birth and abduction. The health care system aims to prevent, detect, and manage human and operational errors. To minimize these errors, the health care staff is trained accordingly so that they can counsel parents. Simultaneously, they will be able to provide emotional support to parents. Both the counseling and emotional support approaches lead to the safety and development of neonates. The trained staffs can ably and closely monitor each newborn baby's condition and respond swiftly to any concerns or emerging issues [23].

Studies observed that the professional midwives trained on Midwife Led Continuity of Care (MLCC) as per the care guidelines that are regulated to international standards can provide better care. Studies show that when the MLCC trained staff supports mothers of newborns, there are 16% less likely chances that the mothers will lose their babies. In addition, the women supported by the MLCC trained staff experience 24% less likely chance to have preterm birth [24].

The section below discusses the importance of food component of the article, which is early initiation of breastfeeding (EIBF) and exclusive breastfeeding (EBF). These two indicators hold good during the first month of life [25].

11. About human Milk

According to the Lancet "human breast milk is a perfectly adapted nutritional supply for the infant. It is probably the most specific personalized medicine that the infant receives at a time when gene expression is being fine-tuned for life" [25].

The importance of EBF can be gauged by the fact that the levels of myo-inositol are high in the first 2 weeks of breastfeeding, and this helps in the wiring of the brain that lays foundation for cognitive development [26].

In order to ensure quality and quantity (Q&Q) of the breast milk, the study advises lactating mothers to have whole grain cereals and seeds as the bran of these foods contains a precursor of inositol called as phytic acid. Almonds, peas, and cantaloupes are foods to be consumed by lactating mothers as these foods are rich sources of inositol [26].

Another study points out that the human milk has an essential nutrient called Docosa Hexanoic Acid (DHA), and Omega-3 fatty acid helps in brain development. The study adds that a severe and fatal gastrointestinal condition called necrotizing enterocolitis (NEC) is prevented by breast milk and probiotics. The intestines of premature babies do not produce enough interleukin (IL) number 22 that protects from microbial infections [27].

12. Literature review

As already discussed above, lower-level health units are the first point of contact for the newborns. A meta-analysis of studies across 44 countries suggests strengthening of these lower-level health units as the main strategy toward reducing neonatal mortality. These units have high caseloads as these are the first point of contacts for the families of newborns. The study concludes on the note that strengthening of such units can yield reduction in mortality rate of newborns [13].

The institutionalized approach comes under the domain of facility-based newborn care (FBNC) that refers to 24*7 services provided by skilled and trained personnel at health facilities. In India at the national level, FBNC started in 1960s in few teaching hospitals or medical colleges. After 40 years, during 1990–2000, Essential Newborn Care (EBNC) that includes activities such as breastfeeding, warmth, and hygiene) was initiated as a strategy. Following this strategy, at the institutional levels newborn care-related equipment such as radiant warmers, resuscitation equipment, weighing scale, and phototherapy units were procured and used. Automatically, training to use these equipment became a regular activity of the FBNC strategy [28–31].

From the national level, efforts were also seen at the subnational levels. In this context, a study in the state of Karnataka showed that research tools, such as supervisory and monitoring checklists, improve the quality of HBNC services. This is a critical area that the current article deals with [32].

Moving further, another study found that FBNC has a component duo called as essential newborn care (EBNC) and sick newborn care (SBNC). The Government of India (GOI) has devised the FBNC guidelines that mention about three levels of newborn care. The first level is at birth, the second level is at the care of normal newborns, and the third level is at the care of sick newborns. These three levels were to be dealt and made operational at the district-level institutional facilities [33].

Like the state of Karnataka, the state of Uttar Pradesh also had a study that elicited the key differences between the FBNC and HBNC. The study explored that use of Ante Natal Care (ANC) and skilled attendance (SA) at the delivery points were strongly associated with Clean Cord Care (CCC) & early initiation of breastfeeding (EIBF). However, the study deduced that the association was not strong with thermal care. Further, the study mentions that in order to maintain thermal care, a symbiotic relationship between HBNC & FBNC is essential [11, 29–31, 34, 35].

As mentioned above, during the 1990–2000 period in India, essential newborn care activities such as breastfeeding, warmth, and hygiene were initiated, conceptualized and put in place at a regular basis. Following this sustained effort, the triad of warmth, food, and security became the triangle of HBNC [36].

A second study in the state of Uttar Pradesh, which is the most populous state of India on HBNC in 2014, brought out the fact that none of the mothers of newborns had adequate knowledge, as well as awareness on the provisions of HBNC. These provisions were for home visits by the ASHAs, and it was observed that the number of home visits by ASHAs to the homes of newborns decreases as the age of the newborn child increases [34].

A study done in 2020 focuses on the dedication of the front line workers (FLWs). The study cites that HBNC is effective in reducing NMR and IMR when delivered by dedicated front line worker (FLW). These are seen not only in community settings but also in institutional settings or newborn care facilities with high rates of facility/institutional births per month/year [29].

Another study threw a perspective on HBNC that deciphers that upscaling of Home-based newborn care (HBNC) needs the support through identification of various limiting factors and effective upscaling in order to enable HBNC for reduction of neonatal mortality (NM) [30].

A 2009 study, which is the third study for the state of Uttar Pradesh in this chapter, reflected that in the parts of Western UP factors, such as awareness and demand for HBNC, were low not only among the mothers but also the community-based service providers, such as ASHAs. The study also mentioned about existing gaps in implementation and roll out of the HBNC strategy [11, 31, 34, 35, 37].

A study also mentions about the obstacles in newborn care, especially the HBNC. The elucidated obstacle was the practice of prelacteal feeding in newborn child. The time limit for prelacteals is the 0–6 days of life. It is to be reinforced that prelacteal feeding (PLF) of the newborns should not be practiced at any cost, and especially it is applicable for the low birth weight (LBW) babies. These LBW babies have birth weight less than 2.5 kilograms. The poor practice of prelacteals feeding (PLF) leads to hypothermia or loss of temperature in the newborn child. The condition of hypothermia leads or aids in infections [18, 31, 34].

The chapter is well served if it mentions studies that deal about causes/determinants of deaths in newborn child out of which infection category leads among all the causes. The section below deals with the fact that occurs if the poor practices, such as pre (0–6 days of life) and post (after 6th day of life) lacteals are not done during the first 28 days of life [11, 35, 37–39].

The current neonatal mortality rate (NMR) in India is 20 per 1000 live births. Similarly, there are multiple benefits of EIBF as well. It reduces the maternal mortality through easing the placental delivery, and thereby the chances of postpartum hemorrhage (PPH) are reduced. Poor practices, such as prelacteal feeding (PLF), happen when unfortunately, maternal mortality (MM) takes place [3, 8].

Another poor practice is the discarding of first breast milk by the lactating mothers. This practice occurs when there is less secretion of breast milk. The less or no secretion of breast milk happens as the newborn child is not put to the breast of the mother, or the EIBF indicator is not adhered to. Communities fall in the trap of these poor religious and cultural practices, while falsely assuming that such practices will help in enhancing the milk secretion in the lactating mothers. The criticality of Colostrum Feeding (CF) or the EIBF indicator is felt when the Maternal Mortality Rate and Ratio (MMR) of India is examined, analyzed and contextualized in the current circumstances at the national and subnational level. Here, it is significant to note that the MM rate in India is 6.0, and the MM ratio is 97 as per the SRS of India. Further, the SRS also mentions that the life time risk (LTR) of a mother in India is 0.3%, which means in probability, out 100 chances, there are 30 chances that the pregnant lady might have a maternal death, assuming that the risk is uniformly distributed along the entire reproductive life of a woman in the reproductive age group of 15–49 years. This high mortality, risk factors, and high death probability can be drastically reduced with the proven and time-tested strategies, such as promotion of EIBF in India and global level. The adoption of EIBF strategy also ensures removal of the two barriers in newborn care [31, 39].

The figure given below is regarding the causes of these neonatal deaths. The figure shows that prematurity is the leading cause among all the categories. In this category, the low birth weight (LBW) babies are included, and the current chapter details out the two barriers/obstacles of the newborns where such LBW babies do not have the strength to suck the breast milk of the lactating mother. The second in line is the neonatal infection (NI) and here the infection prevails because of poor thermal care that leads to hypothermia. It is also critical to note that EIBF is an active component of thermal care as it comes under the domain of Kangaroo Mother Care (KMC). It is proved beyond doubt that timely referrals by FLWs, or family members will definitely help in processes to reduce other causes of neonatal deaths, such as infections and asphyxia. Both FBNC and HBNC roll out have substantiated that hypothermia is a significant contributing factor for such causes that are attributed to neonatal deaths. Hence, the relevance, importance, and timely contextualization of the contents of the current book chapter is clearly in focus in India (**Figure 4**) [39, 41].

A newborn is a boy or girl in the first 4 weeks of life or in the 0–28 days category. India introduced the National Rural Health Mission in 2005. Since the initiation of NRHM across 18 Empowered Action Group (EAG) states, the newborn child care took a paradigm shift. This was because the focus of newborn child care had moved from FBNC to a healthy mix of HBNC and FBNC strategies. The WHO bulletin published in the year 2012 states that India's home-based newborn care (HBNC) model launched in 2011 can be touted as a global policy, and it has percolated to many nations as we can see in 2023 or 12 years after its introduction. The efforts on HBNC were initiated in India in Gadchiroli region of the state of Maharashtra. Here, an effort of 20 years has demonstrated and proved that there was 62% reduction in

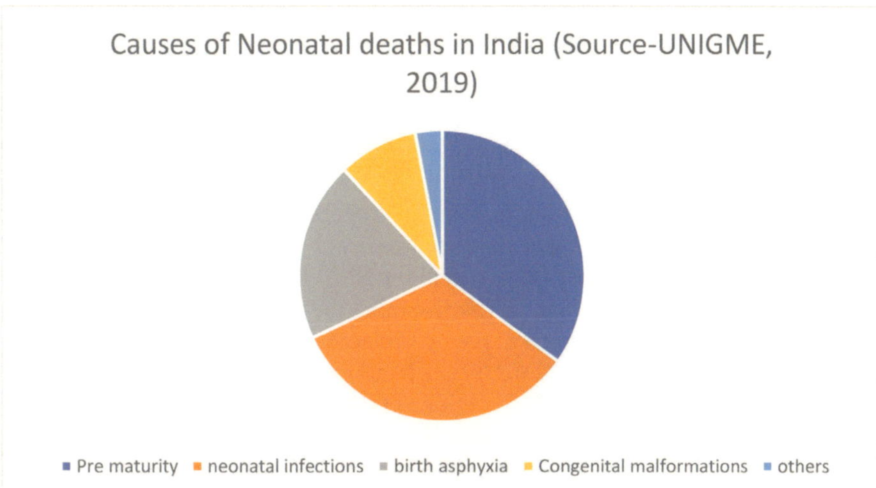

Figure 4.
Causes of neonatal deaths in India [40]—Pie chart by the Lead author.

neonatal mortality through the simple strategy of multiple home visits by community level workers (CLW) [6, 38].

These efforts by the CLWs led to the conceptualization of the NRHM on a large scale at the national level in India in the year 2005. In the strategy of NRHM for newborn care, the FLWs, such as ASHAs, are required to do six home visits to the homes of the new mothers and newborns in case of an institutional delivery and seven home visits in case of a home delivery. Taking the birthday as the "0" day, the visit days for the institutional delivery are on the 3rd, 7th, 14th, 21st,28th, and 42nd days after the delivery. Similarly, the visit days for the home delivery are on the 1st, 3rd, 7th, 14th, 21st, 28th, and 42nd days after birth [6, 8].

When we analyze the pattern of mortality of the newborns, the data regarding weeks showed that 72.9% die in the 0–6-day period. Whereas a mere 13.5% die in the 2nd, 3rd, and 4th weeks after delivery. The neonatal mortality data in percentage per day shows a decreasing trend as the days pass by. There is a difference of 29.5% among o day and day 1 or in just 24 hours. There is an increasing trend between day 1 and day 2. The difference between these 2 days is 2.7%. Thereafter from the 3rd day, the trend shows a continuous decrease. Day wise, the data shows that 36.9% die on day 0, 7.4% on day 1, 10.1% on day 2, 6.6% on day 3, 5.1% on day 4, 3.4% on day 5, and 3.5% on day 6 [42, 43].

Hence, the abovementioned data proves that the first week of life is extremely critical and crucial for the newborn to be visited by the ASHA at the household level. The current chapter focuses on the HBNC model primarily, which is described in detail in the India Newborn Action Plan (INAP) of 2014 of GOI. To augment the home visits by ASHAs, incentivized home-based newborn care program was launched in the year 2011. As on 2023, all the ASHAs of India had been trained as per the training modules of National Health System Resource Centre (NHSRC) of GOI to improve the quality of newborn care services. The figure given below depicts that in the life of an infant, the 1st year of life is critical. In the first year of life, the 1st month of life is more critical. In the first month of life, the 1st week of life is most critical. In the first week of life, the 1st day is utmost critical. In the first day of life, the 1st hour of life is exponentially critical. The triad of activities related to newborn care cannot be missed in the first hour of life or in the first hour after birth as it is known as the golden hour, and it comes once in a life time of the child and does not return again in the life time of the child. Hence, it is re-emphasized that intervening on 1st day and 1st hour is a must [36, 42, 43].

Poor practices, such as prelacteal feed (PLF) and discarding of milk, further increase the risk of the life of the newborn. A related event is that 40% of all stillbirths, and neonatal deaths occur within first 48 hours of life. Further, analysis reflects that about 3/4th of the total neonatal deaths occur in the first week of life or in the 0–6 days period. As mentioned above, 37% of these deaths occur within first 24 hours or on the first day of life. This period is not only critical for NMR but also MMR. During this period, half or 50% of all maternal deaths also takes place. These deaths show the contribution of the poor practices, such as giving prelacteal feeds (PLF) to the newborns. Discarding the first breast milk is done by the lactating mothers who falsely believe that it leads to enhancement of milk secretion. The belief is strong as they the offering is attributed as a religious and cultural practice or taboo [11, 36, 42, 43].

Among the HBNC-related activities, maintaining the warmth component is of utmost importance. Every newborn baby is homoeothermic at birth. From among these newborns, the low birth weight (LBW) babies have decreased thermal insulation as they have reduced amount of brown fat that is situated below the white fat of the skin. The science of matter, physics, tells us that heat loss in the newborn is either due to phenomena such as evaporation, conduction, or convection. Evaporation is through amniotic fluid by surface. Conduction is through touch with cold object or cold skin or body of the caregiver or mother. Convection is through fan or window, where the heavier cold air replaces the lighter warm air. The indicator for the thermal comfort of the newborn child is his or her warm and pink feet. The healthy behaviors such as delayed bathing, delayed weighing, and kangarooing in case of low birth weight (LBW) babies contribute toward maintaining the warmth of the newborn baby. These practices are to be done at both home and institutional level [8, 18, 36].

Moving ahead, maintaining three other components, such as clean airway, breathing and temperature, is also essential in the newborn just like an adult to survive. Above all, the warmth component is of prime importance for low birth weight (LBW) babies because if the LBW babies are not kept warmth, the LBW babies cannot feed and will eventually not gain body weight in the early neonatal period or in the 0–6-day period. To help LBW babies gain weight, timely home visits by ASHAs are not to be missed. The strategy encourages the family members to ensure proper care of the LBW babies there by leading to healthy weight gain in these susceptible LBW babies. It is seen that low-weight neonates are most prone to noncommunicable diseases (NCD) such as diabetes, hypertension, and heart diseases in later life [2–4, 8, 11, 12, 15, 29, 31–35, 44].

13. Neonatal deaths and the modalities

A close look at the analytical epidemiology of deaths of newborns elicits a triad of causes. These are preterm birth complications (PBC) followed by infections. The third cause is intrapartum period related or during delivery. Analysis of the rest of the causes of death shows that there is equal weightage given to congenital anomalies and the "others" category (**Figure 5**) [19, 42, 43].

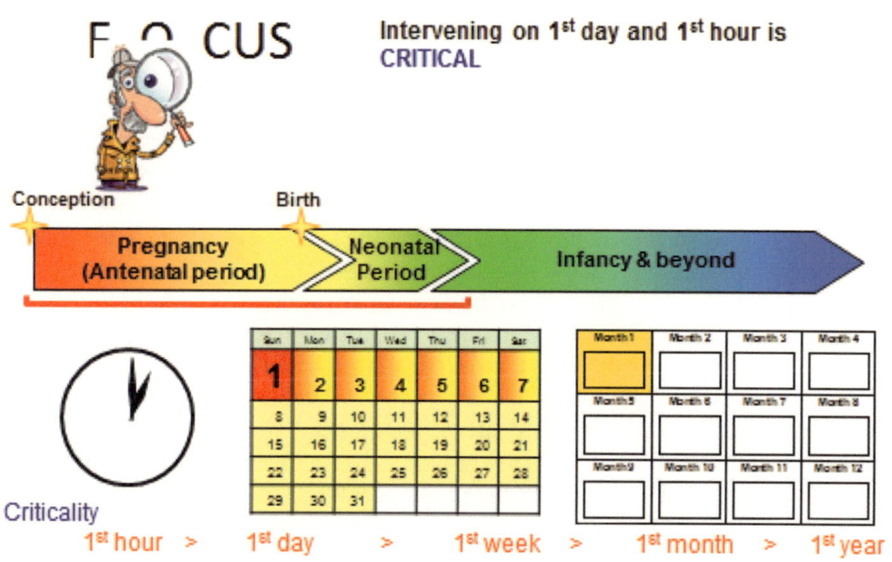

Figure 5.
Critical times of the infancy stage [42, 43]—PowerPoint by the lead author.

The figure given above reiterates the importance of the timing of home visits by ASHAs (Accredited Social Health Activists) in HBNC strategy newborn care. The figure emphasizes that the ASHAs need to plan for the home visits of the newborns. In India, An ASHA covers 1000 population on an average. Hence, at any point of time of the year, there will be 10–12 newborns in her area taking into account the ENMR, LNMR, IMR, abortions and stillbirths (SB) [6, 8].

As mentioned above, when we look at the life risk of the neonate, infant & the U5, we find that among the 1st 5 years of life, 1st year of life is critical. Out of the first 12 months, 1st month is critical. Out of the 1st 4 weeks, the 1st week is critical. Out of the 1st 7 days, the 1st day is critical. Out of the 1st 24 hours, the 1st hour is critical. This 1st at all these levels have a direct relationship with the timing of deaths of the newborns [36, 42, 43].

In India, when we analyze the deaths in weeks, we find that 3/4th of the total neonatal deaths occur in the 1st week of life as discussed above. Among the 1st 7 days of life, the 1st day accounts for more than 1/3rd or 33% as 36.9% of the total neonatal deaths. In other words, the first day deaths are the most critical among the deaths in the entire neonatal period in India at the national level [36, 42, 43].

Further, in another article on neonatal deaths at global level, the lead author M J Shankar deciphers that in the developing countries, the first week of life (0–6 day) period accounts for 77.7% of all neonatal deaths. Further, analysis reflects that 11.1% die in the 2nd week, whereas 11.2% die in 3rd week to 4th week [36, 42, 43].

Epidemiologically, when we the see the deaths in proportions, we find the following proportions of neonatal deaths from among all the neonatal deaths. The proportion in the 1st week of life is given for each of the days of the 1st week in the developing countries [36, 42, 43].

The proportion is 44.4% on day 0. The proportion is 10.1% on day 1. The proportion is 8.3% on day 2. The proportion is 5.8% on day 3. The proportion is 3.6% on day 4. The proportion is 2.7% for days 5 & 6 [36, 42, 43].

Similarly, the same proportion of deaths in India per each day of the 1st week of life shows that on 0 day, the proportion of deaths is 36.9%. The proportion of deaths on 1st day is 7.4%. The proportion of deaths on 2nd day is 10.1%. The proportion of deaths on 3rd day is 6.6%. The proportion of deaths on 4th day is 5.1%. The proportion of deaths on 5th day is 3.4%. The proportion of deaths on 6th day is 3.6% [36, 42, 43].

After seeing the proportion in days, let us see the proportion in weeks. The data reflects that the proportion of deaths in the 1st week is 72.9%. The proportion of deaths in the 2nd to 4th week is 13.5% for each of the 3 weeks [36, 42, 43].

HBNC guidelines are not only regarding newborn care but also on maternal care. It is a package of maternal and child health (MCH0). The guidelines include the care of the mother during pregnancy till 42 days after delivery. To ensure effectiveness of HBNC, during the last trimester of pregnancy, the front line workers (FLWs), such as ASHAs, are expected to visit the homes of the would-be mothers. The discussions of the visits must include appropriate elements of HBNC and the related activities to be done by the household members so that the critical "newborn triad care" is taken care of. As discussed above these are "Warmth,", "Food," and "Security" [4, 8, 36].

During the home visits to the homes of would-be mothers during their last trimester, the FLW should reinforce on four basic activities. These are "wrapping" the newborn immediately after birth, drying the newborn immediately after birth, not bathing the newborn for 7 days after birth and finally giving Kangaroo Mother Care (KMC) to the newborn. All these four activities help maintain the warmth of the child [4, 8, 36].

The FLW should also mention two additional activities during her abovementioned home visit. The activities are giving only colostrums (EIBF) without any pre- and post-lacteals. These activities are to be done in the 0–6-day period. The next activity is exclusive breastfeeding (EBF) the child. Both these activities are toward addressing the food component of the newborn child [4, 8, 36].

Regarding the security aspect, keeping the umbilical cord clean without any application will help prevent Omphalitis. A 24*7 vigil or attending the newborn baby are the activities pointing toward the security needs of the newborn [4, 8, 36].

All the above sections dealt, in the chapter, hope that the objective of the proposed or discussed newborn care approaches is envisaged at a large scale in India. The following section mentions the identification of research gap in the chapter. Addressing this gap will help the country to get optimum output in neonatal care, its positive effect on neonatal care in India and the positive influence it will have in the development of the society and finally its influence on positive trends in framing of newborn friendly health policies in India [6, 41].

Thereafter, the chapter expects that a focused plan to augment and integrate HBNC and FBNC in neonatal health in India is made. It is feasible as it is not only cost effective but also feasible effective as it is done at family or household level without the support of a skilled health provider, such as a clinician/therapeutic provider. It is to be recalled that the HBNC component or the community-level strategy is achieved through the active support of an outreach worker of the public health system, such as the ASHA and the auxiliary nurse midwife (ANM) [3, 8, 11, 12, 15, 32, 40].

14. Identification of research gap

As in any study, the chapter also focuses on the "research gap" following the extensive literature review. The study identifies that outreach approaches of the health systems on EBNC package have not been actively integrated into the entire EBNC package in India. The grassroot level dispensaries of the public health systems work are the "outreach" related stakeholders. These "outreach" centers in fact work vertically, and there is no horizontal integration among the "in-reach" & "outreach" related stakeholders. The integration is especially poor at the community level. The all-important HBNC component is rolled out at this level. As discussed above, the community approaches through the HBNC package roll out have proved its credentials time & again. The credentials are not only in EBNC but also in the field of entire maternal and child health (MCH). Therefore, the research gap concludes that the potential of HBNC has not been actively and appropriately streamlined into the current programmatic interventions on MCH both at subnational and national level in India [12, 24, 28, 32, 33, 35, 37–39].

15. Conclusion

All the elements discussed in the chapter points to the efficacy of the newborn triad of warmth, food, and security. Reduction in NMR is the baseline. If this baseline is taken care of, reduction in IMR and U5MR will eventually happen. As a result, the CMR will reduce which will lead to socioeconomic development through reduction in extreme poverty-stricken families [9, 10, 35, 36].

The normative theory of developmental social policy (DSP) cites that health systems can sustain themselves in the long run. To sustain, health policy (HP) and the health care policy (HCP) paradigm must focus on saving early lives from premature death. Further, lives should be saved from illness, accidents, misery, and poverty. India is adopting the same path of DSP through the various effective and proven strategies on newborn care. It is significant to note that the efforts have percolated across the globe from India, especially on the HBNC strategy of the NHM [11, 45].

Acknowledgements

The lead author wants to acknowledge that Professor Shankar Das, a co-author, was the Ph.D. guide of the lead author at the Tata Institute of Social Sciences (TISS), Mumbai, India during 2011-2018.

Professor D.P.Singh was the teacher of the lead author at TISS, Mumbai during 1995-1997.

The lead author also acknowledges the contributions of all other co-authors.

All the figures given in the chapter have been made by the lead author using the data from the sources mentioned in the chapter against the figures.

Conflict of interest

There is no conflict of interest to write the chapter.

Financial Support

No financial support was received to write the chapter.

Author details

Tridibesh Tripathy[1*], Shankar Das[2], Dharmendra Pratap Singh[3],
Sovesh Chandra Tripathy[4], Anjali Tripathy[5], Sanskriti Tripathy[6], Rakesh Dwivedi[7]
and Mohini Gautam[7]

1 Public Health (Community Medicine) Program, Department of Social Work,
Lucknow University, Lucknow, UP, India

2 School of Health Systems Studies, Tata Institute of Social Sciences, Mumbai, India

3 Centre of Research Methodology, Tata Institute of Social Sciences, Mumbai, India

4 IB Valley Coal Fields, Jharsuguda, Odisha, India

5 LLF, Lucknow, India

6 Bennet University, Greater Noida, Uttar Pradesh, India

7 Department of Social Work, Lucknow University, Lucknow, India

*Address all correspondence to: tridibeshtripathy@gmail.com

References

[1] The Bhagwat Gita. A Scripture of Hindu Mythology. Gorakhpur, Uttar Pradesh, India: Gita Press; 2023

[2] GOI, MOHFW, IIPS, NFHS. GOI, MOHFW, IIPS, NFHS 5 Fact Sheets, 2019-2021. GOI, MOHFW, IIPS. Mumbai, Maharashtra, India: NFHS; 2021

[3] GOI, RGI, SRS, Ministry of Home. Statistical Report, 2020. GOI, Vital Statistics Division, RGI. New Delhi, India: Ministry of Home Affairs; 2022. Available from: http://censusindia.gov.in

[4] GOI, MOHFW, HBNC. GOI, MOHFW, HBNC guidelines. New Delhi, India: GOI, MOHFW, HBNC; 2011

[5] UN, SDG. Goal #3. New York, United States: UN Head Quarters; 2015

[6] NHM. GOI, MCH guidelines. New Delhi, India: NHM; 2007

[7] GOI, NHSRC. Training Modules for ASHAs. New Delhi, India: NRHM; 2005

[8] GOI, MOHFW. India Newborn Action Plan. New Delhi, India: GOI, MOHFW; 2014

[9] GOI. Indian Public Health Standards. New Delhi, India: MOHFW; 2023

[10] Alkire Sabina, Maria Emma Santos. Multidimensional Poverty Index, Oxford Poverty and Human Development Initiative. New York, US: UNDP; 2010

[11] NHM. GOI, MCH guidelines. New Delhi, India: NHM; 2007

[12] GOI, MOHFW. Routine Immunization of India. New Delhi, India: GOI, MOHFW; 2023

[13] Neogi SB et al. Does facility based newborn care improve neonatal outcomes—A review of evidence. Indian Paediatrics. 2012;**49**(8):651-658

[14] GOI, MOHFW. Intensified Mission Indradhanush, Child Health Division. New Delhi, India: GOI, MOHFW; 2023

[15] Neogi SB et al. Inpatient care of small & sick newborns in health care facilities. Journal of Perinatology. 2016;**36**(s3):S18-S23

[16] Sen A et al. Impact of a district level sick newborn care unit on neonatal mortality rate; 2 year follow up. Journal of Perinatology. 2009;**29**:150-155

[17] GOI, MOHFW. IAPPD Guidelines. New Delhi, India: GOI, MOHFW; 2013

[18] National Neonatology Forum teaching aids, new-born care. 2015. Available from: www.nnfi.org/index.php

[19] Liu L et al. National, regional & state level all causes and cause specific U5 mortality in India in 2000-15, a systematic analysis with implications for the SDGs. The Lancet Global Health, Open Access. 2019;**7**(6):e721-e734. DOI: 10.1016/s2214-109x(19)30080-4

[20] Park JE, Park K. Text Book of Preventive & Social Medicine. 11th ed. Jabalpur: M/s Banarasi Bhanot publishers; 1987

[21] Singh M, Saini S. Conceptual Review of Preventive & Social Medicine. 2nd ed. Darya Ganj, New Delhi, India: CBS Publishers & Distributors Pvt. Ltd; 2020. ISBN-978-93-88725-84-2

[22] WHO. Breastfeeding Guidelines. Geneva: WHO; 2022

[23] GOI, MOHFW. National Patient Safety Implementation Framework.

New Delhi, India: GOI, MOHFW; 2018. Available from: https://main.mohfw.gov.in

[24] WHO. Midwifery Education & Care. Geneva, Switzerland: WHO; Available from: https://www.who.int

[25] Victoria C et al. Breast Feeding Series. London, UK: The Lancet; 2016. Available from: https://www.thelancet.com/series/breastfeeding

[26] Biederer T. PNAS study, the importance of myo-inositol in breast milk for baby's brain development. PNAS. 2023;**120**:e2221413120. Available from: www.metroamericas.com/en/noticias-2

[27] Phillips S et al. Global View of Human Milk, GEHM Study. San Diego, CA, United States: PNAS, Neuroscience, University of California; 2021. Available from: www.southeastneo.com/wp-content/uploads/2021

[28] Darnstadt GL et al. Neonatal Survival Series. The Lancet. 2006;**367**(9521):1541-1547

[29] Rasaily R et al. Effect of home based newborn care on neonatal & infant mortality: A cluster randomized trial in India. BMJ Global Health. 2020;**5**:e000680

[30] Dutta AK. Home based newborn care, how effective & feasible? Indian Paediatrics. 2009;**46**:835-840

[31] Baqui AH et al. Newborn Care in Rural Uttar Pradesh. Indian Journal of Paediatrics. 2007;**74**:241-247

[32] Spector JM et al. Improving quality of care in improving maternal & newborn health, prospective pilot study of the WHO safe child birth checklist program. PLoS One. 2012;**7**(5):e35151

[33] Gould JB et al. Expansion of community based perinatal Care in California. Journal of Perinatology. 2002;**22**(8):630-640

[34] Pathak PK et al. Study to assess the HBNC visit in rural areas of Lucnow: A cross-sectional study. Journal of Family Medicine & Primary Care. 2021;**10**(4):1673-1677

[35] Blencowe H, Lee AC, Cousens S, et al. Preterm birth associated neuro developmental impairment estimates at regional and global level for 2010. Paediatric Research. 2013;**74** (Suppl. 1):17-34

[36] Tripathy T et al. FBNC & Homoeopathy. Vol. 12. Issue 07. IJAR. July 2022. pp. 51-54. Print ISSN-2249-555X. 2022

[37] Chaudhury K et al. Deman, awareness & implementation gap of HBNC in rural area of Meerut, UP. IOSR-JDMS. 2019;**18**(6):43-49

[38] Bang AT, Bang RA, Reddy Hanimi M. Home-based neonatal care: Summary and applications of the field trial in rural Gadchiroli, India (1993 to 2003). Journal of Perinatology. 2005;**25**:S108-S122, Nature Publishing Group

[39] GOI, RGI. Vital Statistics Division. New Delhi, India: MMR Bulletin; 2019

[40] UNIGME. Child & Maternal Mortality Division. New York, United States: UNIGME; 2019

[41] UNFPA, NRHM, VHND. UNFPA, NRHM, VHND guidelines. New Delhi, India: UNFPA, NRHM, VHND; 2005

[42] Shankar MJ et al. When do newborns die? A systematic review of timing of overall & cause specific neonatal deaths in developing countries. Journal of Perinatology. 2016;**36**:S1-S11

[43] Shankar MJ et al. State of newborn health in India. Journal of Perinatology. 2016;**36**(Suppl. 3):S3-S8

[44] GOI. GOI, Ministry of H&FW, MCH Guidelines. New Delhi, India: GOI; 2015

[45] Das S, Cottler LB. The health care system in India, chapter 8. In: Aspalter C, Pribadi KT, Gauld R, editors. Health Care Systems in Developing Countries in Asia. 1st ed. UK: Routledge; 2020. ISBN: 9780367594961

Chapter 4

Fight to Survive: An Analysis of the Factors Related to the Control and Elimination of Outbreaks of Multidrug Resistant Bacteria in the Neonatal Intensive Care Units

Santiago Garzón and Fernando Aguinaga

Abstract

The purpose of this chapter is to provide the reader with applicable guidance on the management of outbreaks and infections of multi-resistant bacteria in the neonatal intensive care unit. The main focus will be on the different strategies for the prevention and control of outbreaks of multi-resistant bacteria, these being applied to the personnel and infrastructure of the unit. A brief comparative analysis of different neonatal intensive care units around the world and the similarities and differences in the management of outbreaks and infections will be carried out. The importance of sanitary and epidemiological surveillance and monitoring of outbreaks that can potentially occur in the pediatric intensive care unit, will be addressed in a practical way.

Keywords: neonatal, intensive care unit, multidrug resistant, outbreak, infection, nosocomial

1. Introduction

Neonatal Intensive Care Units represent an environment that must remain relatively free of resistant and multi-resistant pathogens, since this is the area where all newborns coming directly from the delivery room after being in the uterine environment [1].

Outbreaks of bacterial growth, and nosocomial infections acquired in the hospital environment, represent a major global public health problem, having a high frequency in infants hospitalized in the neonatal intensive care area, with a frequency range that varies from 8 to 30%. This data is important, and at the same time alarming, since the mortality and morbidity rate of neonates requiring intensive care increases due to their low immunity, and other associated risk factors such as low birth weight, use of central lines, use of parenteral nutrition, invasive procedures, and early exposure to antibiotics [2, 3].

Mainly, the early and prolonged use of antibiotics, added to the long hospital stays of neonates in intensive care, has allowed a heterogeneous group of resistant and multi-resistant bacteria to cause infectious outbreaks in critical hospital areas.

Among the most important bacteria that cause infectious outbreaks in neonatal intensive care areas we have the *Enterobacteriaceae family,* which are a group of gram-negative, facultative anaerobic bacteria that are saprophytes of the digestive tract, being responsible for between 20% and 40% of late sepsis in neonatal intensive care units [1].

One of the main bacteria in this group is *Klebsiella pneumoniae*, which represents a serious threat to public health, since it is a resistant multidrug bacterium. Other multi-resistant bacteria that occur to a lesser extent, but are the cause of neonatal morbidity and mortality, are *Serratia marcescens*, *Acinetobacter baumanii*, Meticillin-resistant *Staphylococcus aureus*, and vancomycin-resistant enterococcus [4, 5].

The main objective of this chapter is to describe in a practical and didactical way the clinical, epidemiological and microbiological characteristics; and the main intervention measures, to contain or eradicate outbreaks of multi-resistant bacteria in neonatal intensive care units.

2. Determinant measures in the control and elimination of outbreaks of multidrug-resistant bacteria in neonatal intensive care units

The presence of outbreaks of multidrug-resistant bacteria in neonatal intensive care units, and the colonization of hospitalized neonates by those bacteria, is a worrying issue, not only because of the possibility of intestinal or skin colonization, and subsequent hematogenous dissemination causing nosocomial infections; but also, by the chain of transmission of bacteria between health personnel and the environment, creating reservoirs of those bacteria, and multi-resistant genes [1, 3, 6].

The World Health Organization has declared antibiotic resistance in multi-resistant bacteria to be a public health threat, which will have a significant impact on global health, economy and morbidity [7].

Since critically ill neonates are more exposed to being colonized and infected by multi-resistant bacteria mainly due to invasive procedures and antibiotic use, protocols and strategies have been implemented in various neonatal intensive care units worldwide to prevent and eradicate such outbreaks, and its success rate depends on the adherence of the health personnel and the parents of the patients [7, 8].

2.1 Prevention and control measures for outbreaks and infections in neonatal intensive care units

There are several causes that have been investigated as contributing factors to the presence and spread of multi-resistant bacterial outbreaks in neonatal intensive care units [1, 3, 8–10].

Among the main ones, the following have been highlighted:

- Use of powdered neonatal formulas for various patients.
- Use of boiled water, which is not completely sterile.
- Shared use of breast pumps among mothers of infants in the unit.

- Inadequate disinfection of cribs, sinks, and boiled water reservoirs.
- Inadequate hand washing, both by health personnel and parents of patients.
- Ignorance or misapplication of contact isolation protocols in infected or colonized patients.
- Inadequate cleaning and healing of peripheral or central catheters of hospitalized neonates.
- Lack of routine microbiological studies in neonatal intensive care units.

Given the aforementioned causes, some prevention and control measures for outbreaks and nosocomial infections have been implemented. These measures focus on hygiene, timely identification of outbreaks, control of their transmission, and optimization of the proper and conscious use of antibiotics.

2.1.1 Hand hygiene

Hand washing is one of the most important measures to prevent the spread of multi-resistant bacteria. Correct hygiene must be carried out using the 12 steps and the five moments of hand washing established by the World Health Organization (**Figures 1** and **2**).

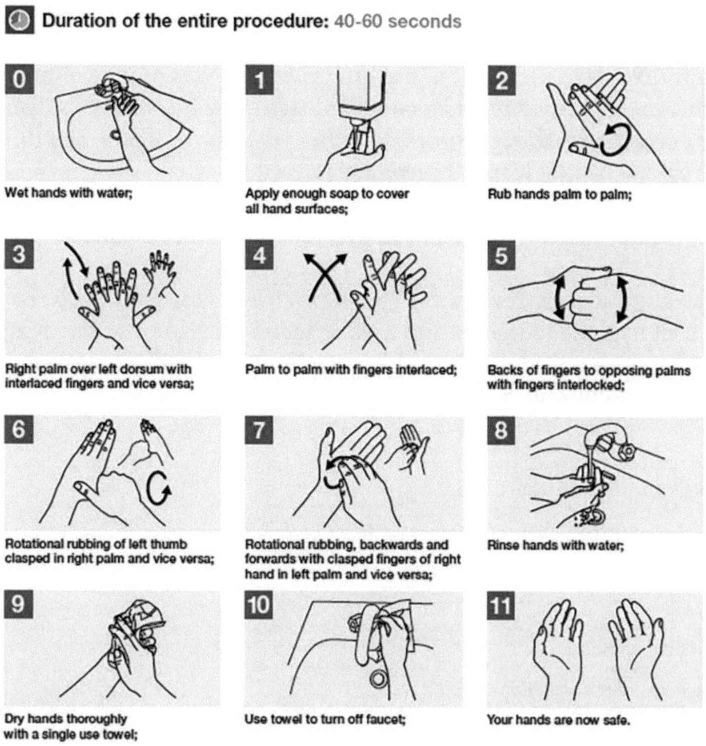

Figure 1.
0–11 steps of hand washing. Under authorization of the WHO [11].

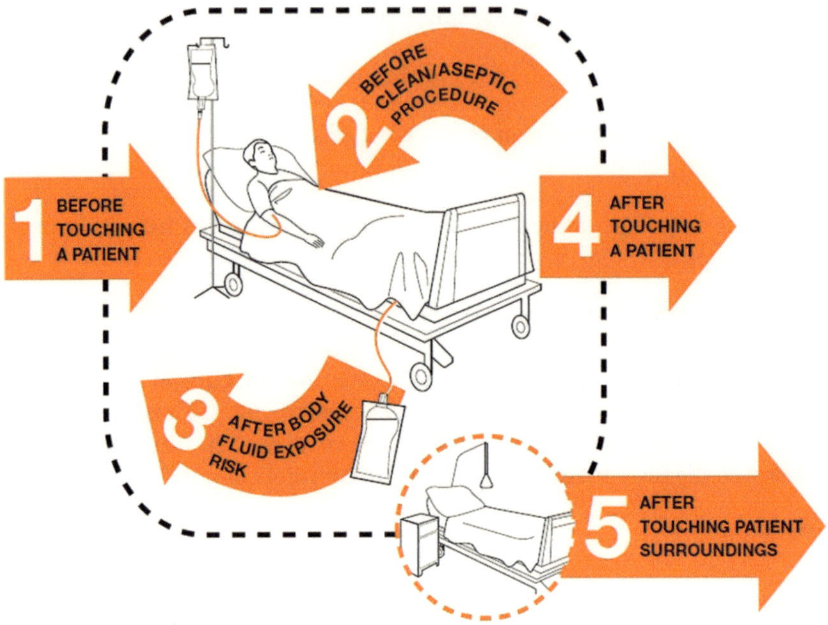

Figure 2.
Five moments for hand hygiene. Under authorization of the WHO [12].

All hand hygiene steps must be performed by both the parents of the neonates, as well as the health and cleaning staff of the neonatal intensive care area.

In the authors experience, a handwashing checklist was implemented in their units (**Table 1**) this checklist that must be complied with by each one of the workers in the neonatology area, and patient visitors, together with the presence of a timer to verify that Hand hygiene lasts at least 40 seconds [1].

2.1.2 Environmental cleaning, medical equipment, and contact isolation

Medium equipment or devices such as respirators or catheters must be used following strict hygiene measures and aseptic techniques for placement and maintenance. In addition, it is very important to carry out regular cleaning and disinfection with appropriate solutions.

Removal of gown, jackets or coats
Removal of rings, watches or bracelets
Sleeve folding
Cap placement
Activation of the stopwatch
Performing the 12 steps of hand washing
Meet the five moments of hand washing

Table 1.
Handwashing checklist. Authorized by the authors [1].

In addition, when an outbreak or infection has been identified in a neonate, he or she should be placed in contact isolation to prevent the transmission and spread of the multiresistant bacteria. This not only implies the physical separation of infected neonates, but the use of individual rooms or cubicles within the infrastructure of the neonatology area.

Disinfectant solutions are used, both in liquid or vaporized form, or in cleaning cloths, containing 17% alcohol solutions, or 35% hydrogen peroxide, or sodium hypochlorite. Those are used for the disinfection of cribs, incubators, medical and nursing equipment, tables, and scales. It is essential that this solutions remains in contact for at least 3 minutes on the area to be disinfected to guarantee a higher success rate [1, 3, 5].

There are several investigations that show a greater advantage in disinfection when it is carried out by direct vaporization of the environment and infrastructure of the unit. The process is simpler, more effective, takes less time, and has a lower degree of toxicity and chemical irritation to the skin of cleaning personnel, health workers, and neonates [3].

2.1.3 Measures that should be implemented in patients in the neonatal intensive care unit

Taking into account that neonatal patients receive breast milk or formula, invasive measures and venous or arterial access are taken, prevention must be carried out in each of these edges to prevent the growth of outbreaks.

A very important measure in neonatal intensive care units is the disinfection and sterilization of the material with which the infant formula is prepared, or the instruments for extracting breast milk, being individualized for each mother of critical neonates. With the respective barrier measures, among which are gloves, gowns, hats and a mask [9, 13].

In addition, it is recommended to use purified water, preferably bottled, for the preparation of formulas; or the use of liquid formulas that are prepared in a sterile manner, discarding the leftovers after their use.

In invasive procedures such as the placement of central lines, venous or arterial access, as well as the disinfection of the entrances of said routes; prior disinfection with 2% chlorhexidine with 0.9% saline solution is recommended, which can be replaced by the use of chlorhexidine sachets [1, 3, 10].

In addition, for the entrances of intravenous devices, the use of caps containing antiseptic substances is recommended.

These infection control measures are very important, since superficial cleaning does not guarantee the eradication of biofilm particles, which can cause cross-transmission of multi-resistant bacteria, with consequent colonization and transmission [4, 9].

2.1.4 Control of visits and effective communication with the newborn's family

Despite the fact that the accompaniment of the family is essential in the recovery of a newborn, it is important to implement restrictions on visits to patients with a more critical condition, since, coming from an environment outside the hospital, they may be carriers of pathogens that can potentially cause outbreaks or infections.

It is a very relevant factor to explain and guide them in a warm and safe way about hand hygiene before and after entering the unit. It must be done under supervision, complying with the hand washing checklist, and putting on gowns and biosecurity measures [9, 10].

2.2 Microbiological characteristics and rational use of antibiotics in neonates

The neonatal intensive care unit is a medical setting in which specialized care is provided to newborns who are premature or seriously ill. The vulnerability of these patients to infections and the importance of adequate treatment makes the rational use of antibiotics a fundamental aspect in clinical practice [8].

2.2.1 Predominant microorganisms

The neonatal intensive care unit is a conductive environment to the proliferation of bacteria, fungi, and other pathogens.

Some of the more common bacteria include *Staphylococcus aureus*, *Escherichia coli*, *Klebsiella pneumoniae*, and Enterobacter spp. In addition, fungi of the Candida species are an important cause of infections in neonates [1, 8].

2.2.2 Antimicrobial resistance

Frequent exposure to antibiotics in the neonatal intensive care unit has led to the development of antimicrobial resistance to pathogens. This complicates treatment and increases the morbidity of newborns [9, 10, 14].

The colonization of neonates with multi-resistant bacteria is a worrying issue for public health, not only because of the possibility of a serious nosocomial infection, but also because of the creation of reservoirs of multi-resistant bacteria and bacterial resistance genes.

Various mechanisms of bacterial resistance have been developed, such as the production of extended-spectrum beta-lactamases, and the production of carbapenemases. All this, coupled with poor control of antibiotic management, neonatal immunological immaturity, and invasive procedures in neonates, make the impact on prognosis, hospital stay, and hospital costs greater [1].

2.2.3 Empirical therapy and rational use of antibiotics

Early and accurate diagnosis of an infection is essential for the rational use of antibiotics. Appropriate microbiological and diagnostic tools such as blood cultures, cerebrospinal fluid analysis, and antibiotic susceptibility testing should be used [1, 15].

Since the results of culture results can take several days, it is common for empiric antibiotic therapy to be started. However, this therapy should be based on local knowledge of resistance patterns and adjusted based on culture results and susceptibility testing [1, 7, 15].

Antibiotics must be given for as long as necessary to treat the infection. As soon as possible, de-escalation should be considered, that is, adjusting the treatment according to the results of the cultures and the clinical stay of the patient, thus avoiding unnecessary and prolonged exposure to antibiotics [1, 7, 9].

2.3 Education and training of health personnel

The education of health personnel must include a solid understanding of antimicrobial resistance and its clinical implications.

Training should be carried out on adequate hygiene practices, such as correct hand washing, the correct use of personal protective equipment, and cleaning and disinfection of surfaces and equipment. In addition, they must be aware of infection control policies and protocols [1, 3].

Education and training should foster interdisciplinary collaboration in the neonatal intensive care unit. This implies effective communication between doctors, nurses, microbiologists and other health professionals involved in the care of newborns [9, 15].

2.4 Importance of epidemiological surveillance

Epidemiological surveillance refers to the systematic collection, analysis and interpretation of data related to the health of the population. In our context, their intervention in the neonatal intensive care unit implies constant monitoring of the appearance of infections and the identification of patterns to prevent the spread of multi-resistant bacteria [1, 6].

It plays a fundamental role in the prevention and control of outbreaks of multi-resistant bacteria. These outbreaks are a significant threat to the health of sick and premature newborns, and can have serious and even fatal consequences [1, 6].

2.4.1 Early surveillance of outbreaks and implementation of control measures

Early surveillance of outbreaks allows the detection of multi-resistant bacteria. By continuously monitoring infection data, unusual increases in infection incidence can be identified and preventative measures taken before it becomes uncontrollable [1, 2, 6].

In addition, through timely surveillance, control measures for the prevention and spread of outbreaks can be quickly implemented.

These measures may include the adoption of stricter hygiene practices, the promotion of vaccination, the optimization of the use of antibiotics and the segregation of infected patients [1, 2, 6].

It is essential to carry out microbiological studies, processing specific cultures of neonatal patients, and their environment, such as sinks, cribs, hands of medical and nursing staff, and boiled water reservoirs and formula cans [1, 4, 16].

2.4.2 Monitoring the effectiveness of interventions

The continuous monitoring of the established interventions allows tracking the results of the control measures, in this way it can be determined if they are having the desired impact in the reduction of outbreaks of multi-resistant bacteria. This provides an opportunity to adjust and improve prevention strategies [1, 3].

In addition to the detection of multi-resistant bacteria, epidemiological surveillance of the neonatal intensive care unit plays a key role in monitoring antimicrobial resistance. This helps identify patterns of resistance and guide the appropriate selection of antibiotics for the treatment of neonatal infections [1, 3, 10].

3. Analysis of success stories

In the authors' experience, a strategy to eradicate an outbreak of Carbapenemase-producing *Klebsiella pneumoniae* was implemented in the neonatology area of a hospital in Ecuador.

It was observed that, by implementing and educating about the handwashing checklist, a 99% adherence to the five moments and 12 steps of handwashing could be seen. This was applied both to medical personnel and to the relatives of the neonates who stayed with them, thus demonstrating that the main control measure was education for health personnel working in the neonatology area [1].

Several serial cultures were carried out, decreasing their positivity, noting in the long term that the establishment of the measures reduced the presence of the outbreak until its complete eradication after 1 year of follow-up [1].

Several similar studies carried out in Colombia, Italy, and Spain implemented a package of similar measures, with certain changes, such as daily bathing of patients with chlorhexidine gluconate, and monthly monitoring of the outbreak with cultures [1, 17].

In a neonatal intensive care unit in Australia, after presenting an outbreak of multi-resistant gram negative bacteria, the removal of sinks and a change in the neonatal bathing strategy were implemented as a strategy. They showed that the cessation of the daily bathing routine for neonates, and changing and cleaning the sinks consistently reduced the outbreak, emphasizing the need to control and treat water in neonatal units [6].

In a study carried out in Brazil, they observed that the extended use of antibiotics in neonatal patients was associated with the presence of multi-resistant bacteria, focusing on the rational use of antibiotics as a measure to reduce outbreaks in the neonatal intensive care unit [2].

In Malaysia, an outbreak of *Acinetobacter baumanii* was successfully eradicated from a neonatal intensive care unit. The researchers showed that poor hand washing, lack of disinfection of supplies and poor storage of breast milk and infant formulas were the source of colonization and the presence of the outbreak. They implemented a systematic check-up to control hand washing, sink cleaning, good management of breast milk storage, and control of neonatal hygiene, with which they managed to contain the outbreak [15].

In France, an outbreak of *Enterobacter cloacae* was investigated in a neonatal intensive care unit, implementing contact isolation measures, sterilization of breast milk pumps, reduction of the use of broad-spectrum empirical antibiotic therapy, and education of health personnel [9].

4. Challenges faced by neonatal intensive care units

Neonatal intensive care units face several challenges in the fight against multi-resistant bacteria due to the vulnerability of newborns and the complexity of the hospital environment. The most common challenges include:

- Limited immunity: critically ill or premature infants in intensive care often have immature or weakened immune systems, making them more susceptible to bacterial infections, primarily nosocomial ones. In addition, they often require invasive procedures and broad-spectrum antimicrobial therapy, further increasing the risk of multidrug-resistant infections [10, 17].

- Cross transmission: neonatal intensive care units are environments with a high density of patients and staff, which facilitates the transmission of multi-resistant bacteria between sick neonates. Germs can spread through direct or indirect contact, such as medical equipment, staff's hands, the air, and water [3, 13].

- Inappropriate use of antibiotics: the excessive or inappropriate use of antibiotics in neonatal intensive care units can favor the development and spread of multi-resistant bacteria. This can occur when antibiotics are prescribed without adequate assessment for infection or when broad-spectrum therapies are used without adequate monitoring [9, 14].

- Diagnostic limitations: early and accurate identification of bacterial infections in newborns can be complicated due to the lack of specific symptoms and the difficulty in obtaining quality laboratory specimens. This can delay proper treatment and facilitate the spread of multi-resistant bacteria [4, 10].

5. Conclusions and recommendations

Although the management of multi-resistant bacteria in the Pediatric Intensive Care area can be a complex challenge, it is possible to address it taking into account the premises of this chapter and applying them in the different areas of intensive care, not only neonatal, but also pediatric and adult.

The key is in the adoption of strict prevention measures, in order to promote a culture of health safety and health awareness in all health personnel, and the parents of newborns who are a key part in their recovery.

The multidisciplinary approach in the fight against multi-resistant bacteria in the pediatric intensive care unit must involve not only doctors and nurses, but also microbiologists, epidemiologists, and different public health coordination areas. This will allow you to create more effective strategies and with a greater focus.

Active surveillance of infections and outbreaks, continuous monitoring of bacterial resistance, and rational use of antibiotics are crucial measures to prevent the emergence and spread of multi-resistant bacteria. This involves systematic data collection and analysis, careful assessment of the need for antibiotics, selection of specific and targeted therapies for each patient and identified pathogen, optimal duration of treatment, as well as implementation of follow-up and feedback programs to assess the effectiveness of interventions.

Another important pillar is continuous education and training for staff on the best infection prevention and control practices. In addition to creating awareness in each of the importance of hand hygiene, rational use of antibiotics, early identification of outbreaks. A fundamental part of education is effective communication with parents, instructing them on biosafety standards when entering to see their children.

Continuous education, involving both family members and health personnel are very important and fundamental pillars to reduce the incidence of outbreaks and infections, and thus reduce their impact on the care units. Neonatal intensive care, and decrease neonatal mortality.

Conflict of interest

The authors declare no conflict of interest.

Thanks

The authors thank their neonatal patients who tirelessly fight every day to get ahead.

We thank our families and neonatology for being passionate every day to give the best for the benefit of newborns.

Author details

Santiago Garzón* and Fernando Aguinaga
Hospital Metropolitano, Quito, Ecuador

*Address all correspondence to: santi_garzon@hotmail.com

References

[1] Garzón S, Ullauri J, Aguinaga F, Flores K. Factors related to the control and elimination of an outbreak of Carbapenemase producing *Klebsiella pneumoniae* in the Neonatology Unit of the Hospital Metropolitano de Quito. Revista Ecuatoriana de Pediatria. 2020;**21**:1-11. Article 14. DOI: 10.52011/0027

[2] Baek EH, Kim SE, Kim S, Lee S, Cho OH, In Hong S, et al. Successful control of an extended-spectrum beta-lactamase-producing *Klebsiella pneumoniae* ST307 outbreak in a neonatal intensive care unit. BMC Infectious Diseases. 2020;**20**(1):1-8. DOI: 10.1186/s12879-020-4889-z

[3] Bustos-Moya G, Josa-Montero D, Perea-Ronco J, Gualtero-Trujillo S, Ortiz-Aroca J, Novoa-Bernal Á, et al. Factors related to the successful control of an outbreak caused by KPC-2-producing Klebsiella pneumoniae in an intensive care unit in Bogotá, Colombia. Infection. 2016;**20**(1):25-32. DOI: 10.1016/j.infect.2015.07.001

[4] Chen D, Hu X, Chen F, Li H, Wang D, Li X, et al. Co-outbreak of multidrug resistance and a novel ST3006 *Klebsiella pneumoniae* in a neonatal intensive care unit: A Retrospective study. Medicine. United States. 2019;**98**(4):1-7. DOI: 10.1097/MD.0000000000014285

[5] Fernández-Prada M, Martínez-Ortega C, Santos-Simarro G, Morán-Álvarez P, Fernández-Verdugo A, Costa-Romero M. Outbreak of extended-spectrum beta-lactamase-producing *Klebsiella pneumoniae* in a neonatal intensive care unit: Risk factors and key preventive measures for eradication in record time. Annals of Pediatric. 2019;**91**(1):13-20. DOI: 10.1016/j.anpedi.2018.06.021

[6] Tracy M, Ryan L, Samarasekara H, Leroi M, Polkinghorne A, Branley J. Removal of sinks and bathing changes to control multidrug-resistant gram-negative bacteria in a neonatal intensive care unit: A retrospective investigation. Journal of Hospital Infection. 2020;**104**(4):508-510. DOI: 10.1016/j.jhin.2020.01.014

[7] Saporito L, Graziano G, Mescolo F, Amodio E, Insinga V, Rinaudo G, et al. Efficacy of a coordinated strategy for containment of multidrug-resistant gram-negative bacteria carriage in a neonatal intensive care unit in the context of an active surveillance program. Antimicrobial Resistance and Infection Control. 2021;**10**(1):1-12. DOI: 10.1186/s13756-021-00902-1

[8] Gülsoy Z, Karagozoglu S. The efficiency of cleaning in intensive care units: A systematic review. Enfermeria Intensiva. 2022;**33**(2):92-106. DOI: 10.1016/j.enfi.2021.02.002

[9] Rahal A, Andreo A, Le Gallou F, Bourigault C, Bouchand C, Ferriot C, et al. Enterobacter cloacae complex outbreak in a neonatal intensive care unit: Multifaceted investigations and preventive measures are needed. Journal of Hospital Infection. 2021;**116**(2021):87-90. DOI: 10.1016/j.jhin.2021.07.012

[10] Ababneh Q, Abulaila S, Jaradat Z. Isolation of extensively drug resistant *Acinetobacter baumannii* from environmental surfaces inside intensive care units. American Journal of Infection Control. 2022;**50**(2):159-165. DOI: 10.1016/j.ajic.2021.09.001

[11] World Health Organization. Your 5 Moments for Hand Hygiene. 2009. Available from: https://cdn.who.int/media/docs/

default-source/integrated-health-services-(ihs)/infection-prevention-and-control/your-5-moments-for-hand-hygiene-poster.pdf?sfvrsn=83e2fb0e_21

[12] World Health Organization. How to handwash? 2009. Available from: https://www.who.int/docs/default-source/patient-safety/how-to-handwash-poster.pdf?sfvrsn=7004a09d_2

[13] Chiguer M, Maleb A, Amrani R, Abda N, Alami Z. Assessment of surface cleaning and disinfection in neonatal intensive care unit. Heliyon. 2019;**5**(12):e02966. DOI: 10.1016/j.heliyon.2019.e02966

[14] Agyepong N, Fordjour F, Owusu-Ofori A. Multidrug-resistant *Acinetobacter baumannii* in healthcare settings in Africa. Frontiers in Tropical Diseases. 2023;**4**:1-9. DOI: 10.3389/fitd.2023.1110125

[15] Woon JJ, Ahmad Kamar A, Teh CSJ, Idris N, Zhazali R, Saaibon S, et al. Molecular epidemiological investigation and management of outbreak caused by carbapenem-resistant *Acinetobacter baumannii* in a neonatal intensive care unit. Microorganisms. 2023;**11**(4):1-11. DOI: 10.3390/microorganisms11041073

[16] Weinberg SE, Villedieu A, Bagdasarian N, Karah N, Teare L, Elamin WF. Control and management of multidrug resistant *Acinetobacter baumannii*: A review of the evidence and proposal of novel approaches. Infection Prevention in Practice. 2020;**2**(3):100077. DOI: 10.1016/j.infpip.2020.100077

[17] Escobar, Pérez JA, Olarte Escobar NM, Castro-Cardozo B, Valderrama Márquez IA, Garzón Aguilar MI, De La Barrera LM, et al. Outbreak of NDM-1-producing *Klebsiella pneumoniae* in a neonatal unit in Colombia. Antimicrobial Agents and Chemotherapy. 2013;**57**(4):1957-1960. DOI: 10.1128/AAC.01447-12

Section 2

Essential Practices in Neonatal Care

Chapter 5

Noise: The Importance of Silencing the Loud NICU

Vita Boyar and Annmarie Gennattasio

Abstract

In utero, the growing fetus is subject to low-frequency noises. However, the high-risk neonate experiences much harsher sounds in the extrauterine environment. Despite many advances, modern Neonatal Intensive Care units cannot mimic the womb environment for preterm infants. Neonates are exposed to a stressful noisy environment where sleep is frequently interrupted and physiologic consequences alter development. Undesirable noise can be generated from simple conversation, use of equipment, overhead announcements, surrounding objects, and vibration. Noise levels above the American Academy of Pediatrics (AAP) recommendation (under 35–45 decibels [dB]) are associated with adverse outcomes and hearing loss. Noise level in the NICU is an important patient safety issue and should be regularly addressed by healthcare providers. Understanding modifiable and non-modifiable noise can influence daily practices, NICU design, staff education, and unit-specific quality improvement programs.

Keywords: noise reduction, preterm infants, acoustic development, neurodevelopment, staff education, neonatal unit, devices, parents as partners

1. Introduction

In utero, the growing fetus is subject to low-frequency noises. However, the high-risk neonate experiences much harsher sounds in the extra uterine environment [1]. The Neonatal Intensive Care Unit (NICU) is a place, in theory, that should mimic the womb for preterm infants. However, the NICU is a stressful environment where sleep is frequently interrupted by procedures and loud unpredictable noises. Undesirable and excessive noise results from medical activities, monitor alarms, conversations, and visitors. Calikusu-Incekar and Balci [1] reported that the two biggest sources of noise in the NICU are monitor alarms and human voices. In addition, NICU architecture, devices used and the type of incubator may determine a neonate's exposure to noxious sounds [2–5].

The American Academy of Pediatrics (AAP) recommends limiting noise in the NICU to <45 decibels [dB] and states that exposure to higher noise levels can have deleterious effects on high-risk newborns [3, 6–9]. Noise can cause alterations in blood pressure, heart rate, and respiratory rate [8]. Due to impaired autoregulation of cerebral perfusion in preterm neonates, these fluctuations can contribute to intraventricular hemorrhage (IVH) and cerebral ischemia [10, 11]. Grades 3 and 4 IVH are associated with neurodevelopmental delays [12].

IntechOpen

Noise exerts stress on both infants and staff in the NICU. For infants, stress from noise increases the consumption of calories and disrupts normal growth and development [6, 13]. These can contribute to increased length of NICU stay, more need for rehabilitative care, and increased health care costs [14]. For staff, excessive noise stress is associated with suboptimal performance and job burnout [3, 5, 6, 14–17].

Nevertheless, noise levels in NICU regularly exceed 45 dB and often rise to levels as high as 120 dB. Several approaches have been reported to promote a "culture of silence," including quiet time protocols, staff education programs, visual noise feedback monitors, and staff "sound compliance supervisors" [5, 18–21]. Ongoing staff education programs, coupled with monitoring noise levels, are essential to sustaining a commitment to noise reduction in the NICU. Parents and family members can also be supported to engage in developmentally appropriate care to become competent caregivers and advocates for the neuroprotection of their babies [22, 23]. Quiet time protocols may significantly decrease exposure to electronic sounds and voices, increasing restful sleep and promoting growth [5, 24]. In contrast, some other interventions, such as the use of earmuffs, do not have clear benefits [25–27].

The physiologic consequence of unpredictable loud sounds and the negative effect on neonatal growth and development is a clinical concern and an important patient safety issue that should be regularly addressed by healthcare providers.

2. What is noise?

Sound encompasses everything we can hear, while noise is characterized as undesirable sound or disturbing sound often linked to its volume [28–30]. Noise has also been described as that which exceeds the human auditory tolerance thresholds [31]. Undesirable noise has been associated with negative long-term impacts on humans, other forms of life, and biodiversity, leading to approximately 1 million disability-adjusted life-years lost each year in Western Europe, as estimated by The World Health Organization (WHO). Noise can cause direct injury to the auditory system causing hearing impairment, tinnitus, increased incidence of cardiovascular diseases, disturbed sleep patterns, and impaired cognitive performance [29].

Four primary types of noise have been described: continuous, sporadic, impulsive, and low-frequency. Continuous noise is sound that has the same frequency, volume, and quality, uninterrupted over time remaining stable and constant. Sporadic noise also referred to as intermittent or variable, tends to be inconsistent, increasing and decreasing rapidly. Impulsive noise can be defined as impact noise in which extremely short bursts of loud sounds last for short durations of time. Low-frequency noise is the faint background soundscape humming or buzzing emitted from equipment, electronic devices, and ventilation systems [30, 31].

Noise can also be described in terms of colors. Each color is defined denoting a specific frequency of sound wave. High-frequency sounds are perceived as higher pitched and low-frequency sounds are lower pitched. There are many different hues of noise but the most well-known and studied are white, pink, and brown noises [32].

Humans perceive different types of noise based on the number of times the sound waves repeat per second. White noise contains every frequency that a human ear can hear, spanning 20–20,000 Hertz (Hz) (a unit measuring frequency, equal to one cycle per second [33]). This range of noise frequencies is fast and random similar to radio static. Pink noise is a more balanced spectrum than white, dampening the volume of higher frequencies resembling steady rainfall or a mother's heartbeat heard by a fetus in the womb. Brown noise further suppresses high frequencies, creating deeper masking sounds, such as distant thunder, drawing inspiration from Brownian motion, the random movement of microscopic particles suspended in liquid or gas [32, 34].

2.1 Measurements of noise

Noise levels are quantified using Sound Pressure Level (SPL), expressed in decibels (dB). SPL represents the amplitude, strength, or force of a sound wave [35], measuring the difference between the sound wave pressure and the ambient pressure of what the sound is traveling through. Sound pressure level uses Pascal's initially as its unit of measurement then is converted into the decibel scale. This conversion helps give a numerical value to noise and helps to define acceptable levels to prevent hearing loss and other noise-related health concerns. The dB scale is logarithmic. For example, if a sound registers 80 dB, it is 10 times more intense than 70 dB. The A-weighted decibels (dBa) measurement is commonly used when measuring sound for healthy versus unhealthy levels. A-weighted decibels consider the human ear's sensitivity to sound intensity, different frequencies, and how the human ear responds whereas dB is based only on sound intensity [36–38].

3. Developing neonate and noise exposure

Preterm birth interrupts the normal physiologic developmental pattern of many organs and introduces external conditions necessitating adaptation and alternate maturational processes that can be detrimental to neonates' maturation and long-term developmental outcomes. Fetal avoidance of noxious stimuli is supported by in-utero mechanisms. The developing fetus is protected from trauma by cushioning amniotic fluid, infection by amniotic membranes, malnutrition by placental nutrient transfer, and excessive light and noise by layers of amniotic fluid and maternal structures. The first sounds the fetus is exposed to are maternal heartbeat, digestive sounds, and muffled outside noises. These sounds are transmitted via bone conduction and fluid medium, as the air conduction system is not developmentally mature until close to full term [39]. The majority of sounds transmitted to fetuses are low-frequency (<500 Hz) positive sounds (human language) and periodic, rhythmic, and even predictable sounds (e.g.: heartbeat). Structural components of the inner ear (labyrinth and cochlear) are formed by 15 weeks but are not functional until 24–25 weeks gestation. Electrophysiologic data [39, 40] demonstrates preterm brainstem evoked potentials between 25 and 32 weeks. At this time the hearing threshold is around 40 dB [41]. Before 27 weeks gestation no fetuses respond to higher frequencies (>500 Hz). After 34 weeks gestation age (GA), the spiral ganglion neurons and cochlea have adequate neural connections that evolve and populate the path toward the auditory cortex. Responses to higher frequencies (>1000 Hz) are observed after 34 weeks. GA, as speech patterns are recognizable and learning and memory formations begin [41, 42]. Development of the inner cells of the cochlea is a pre-determined, ordered process with specific topography of hair cells. This topography ensures the maturation of "low-frequency" regions first, protecting neurons from high-frequency injury as they are mildly unresponsive to random, high-frequency sounds. This process is referred to as "frequency-dependent plasticity" and is imperative to prevent injury to developing structures.

As pregnancy progresses maternal structures and tissues thin out and higher-frequency sounds are gradually transmitted through. There is a preference for naturalistic sounds such as voice recognition, vowel discrimination, and soft classical music [5, 24, 43, 44]. Interruption of physiologic topographic maturity and exposure to developmentally inappropriate frequencies injures migrating neurons, hair cells, and cochlea fluid composition, leading to cell injury, inflammation, and eventually poor frequency resolution, hearing loss, and stressful response to noises leading to systemic manifestations [44, 45]. These findings have been demonstrated in animal studies upon exposure to poor-quality, random, high-frequency noise. These models revealed malformed topographic maps, injured neurons and supportive cells, inflammation, and premature neuronal firing culminating in decreased hearing quality and accelerated age-related hearing loss [39, 45].

3.1 Short-term pathologic changes in responses to noise

Noise levels above the recommendations (under 35–45 decibels (dB)) as determined by the AAP, the World Health Organization (WHO), and the Environmental Protection Agency (EPA) are associated with alterations in vital signs, such as blood pressure, heart rate and respiratory rate [3, 6, 8, 13–15, 28, 46–48].

3.1.1 Heart rate (HR)

Exposure to high-frequency noise has been shown to elicit inappropriate tachycardia in neonates. Preterm babies may not be able to compensate for prolonged tachycardia, leading to bradycardia and altered oxygen delivery. Blood pressure (BP) fluctuations may follow, leading to the transmission of inappropriate blood pressure to cerebral vasculature via passive cerebral circulation and increased risk of intraventricular hemorrhage [48]. The cardiac response to loud noise depends on a history of previous noise exposure, habituation with exposure, behavioral state and integrity of the central nervous system, other insults, and gestation age.

3.1.2 Respiratory rate (RR)

Loud noise induces tachypnea, interfering with normal oxygen delivery to the tissues. Studies have demonstrated decreased oxygen saturation both in awake and sleep states [3]. Other studies noted decreased respiratory rate to pathologic levels, especially with very loud (100 dBA) frequencies [48].

3.1.3 Growth

Studies demonstrated an increase in intracranial pressure and changes in electromyography readings during HR and BP fluctuations due to noise. Interestingly, the changes negatively affect the neuroendocrine system as well as the immune system [6]. Stress activates the hypothalamic-pituitary-adrenal axis and causes growth-inhibiting effects, likely via corticosteroid action [6, 10, 11].

Changes in HR, RR, and oxygen saturation demand increased caloric expenditure. Preterm neonates, in particular, have immature mechanisms for calming themselves and compensating. Prolonged noise exposure leads to poor growth, prolonged stay in the NICU, and delayed acquisition of feeding skills [3]. Investigators have tried to minimize the exposure to noise by providing earmuffs or silicone earplugs. The conclusion is not clear, as some studies show increased stress from just wearing the muffs and others show a decrease in noise transmission without any meaningful physiologic improvement [3]. At this point, universal earmuffs are not recommended for preterm neonates [49].

3.1.4 Impaired sleep

Physiologic habituation to noise is impaired in preterm neonates leading to diminished rapid eye movement (REM) and non-REM sleep. Sleep deprivation can lead to fatigue, agitation, irritability, and even increased intracranial pressure. During the non-REM stage of sleep brain maturation as relates to neurodevelopment takes place. Cerebellum, midbrain, hippocampus, and brainstem growth, differentiation, and synaptogenesis take place mostly during sleep. Reducing noise and light allows the longest and the best quality of sleep [19]. Some studies do show longer sleep in babies provided earplugs or muffs [3]. Some report improved weight gain and greater head circumference, but the numbers are not sufficient to show consistent clinical significance, and more studies are needed. Research suggests that periods of prolonged (at least 90 minutes) quiet time is required to observe meaningful physiologic differences [19].

3.1.5 Perception and response to pain stimuli

Noise diminishes the ability to soothe oneself and tolerate pain. The pathologic response is a disordered neuronal firing, leading to further irritability, crying, and systemic physiologic dysregulation. Repeat stimulation leads to maladaptive behaviors, exaggerated pain, and a startle response. As the topography of neonatal neuronal pain pathways is developing, the long-term responses show hyperactivity, inability to "center" oneself, and exaggerated stress response to future minor stimuli [39, 41, 42].

3.2 Long-term neurodevelopment sequelae

As an infant matures early exposure to caustic noise diminishes linguistic efficiency. Preterm birth switches pre-programmed in-tuning to sound of voice to harmful background noise, that normally would be filtered. Immaturity of the negative feedback leads to over-processing of the pervasive noise, training the immature preterm brain to over-emphasize high-frequency noise that competes with positive speech sounds. In addition, polluting background noises muffle out beneficial speech, leading to delays in language acquisition. Lack of long periods of parental presence in the NICU and exposure to their speech leads to relative "silence" of memory-producing teachable phonetics, despite surrounding caustic noise, leading to hearing deprivation. Likely auditory plasticity persists throughout life and appropriate training can improve language acquisition and clarity [3, 12, 19, 48].

4. Noise–Where does it come from?

Noise can be generated from simple conversation, use of equipment, overhead announcements, vibration from electronic equipment, ventilators, infusion pumps, vital sign monitors, blood pressure machines, suction machines, portable radiograph machines, ultrasound equipment, dragging chairs, isolettes, and extracorporeal membrane oxygenation (ECMO) systems [28].

Emergencies, procedure times, response time to silencing alarms, change of shift reporting, bedside provider rounds, and family visiting all impact the level of noise in the NICU. These sources of noise have been linked to spikes in noise levels and have been barriers to successful noise reduction programs. Other factors contributing to the elevated noise levels in the NICU include healthcare providers talking in loud conversational voices at the bedside and not promptly silencing the monitor alarms, the number of people in the patient room, the number of neonates in the room, the number of alarms activated, infant acuity, and the work-shift type [50, 51]. Staff and visitors' general attitudes have also been identified as a main source of noise. In one study, conversation constituted 50% of the noise-producing sources. A high number of healthcare professionals, a high patient census, and numerous visitors at any given time are also associated with a significant increase in noise levels. Other sources are the use of telephones, oxygen and compressed air sources, humidifiers, and suction machines. Unwanted harsh increases in noise levels are also produced by overhead announcements and fire alarm notifications. Increased unwanted noise has also stemmed from aging NICU and housekeeping equipment but also from newer electronic equipment such as motion-sensor paper towel dispensers or newer staff communication devices [45].

Neonatal incubators serve as a home to neonates in a NICU for prolonged periods. Modern incubators are advanced, microprocessor-controlled, double plexiglass wall units that utilize special quiet technology. Despite modern advances, the noise level within the incubator varies between 55 and 70 dB. contributing significantly to hearing insults despite theoretically providing partial protection from outside noise [38, 44, 52]. In addition, due to reverberance effects, the incubator amplifies the internal noise produced by the cooling fan as well as magnifies the intensity of the baby's cry. The cooling fan is known to produce tones at 200, 400, and 600 Hz, which if eliminated could decrease the noise by 4–6 dB. Studies have shown transmission of even higher frequencies through the open doors, lack of incubator protective effects of noise with respiratory equipment in use, and almost zero effect of incubator covers [47, 49]. In addition, incubators boost transmission of low frequencies (below 125 Hz) due to strong resonance [14]. Other incubator-associated activities such as closing doors generate a sound of 85 dB, placing an object on the incubator emits 90 dB, and closing the lower drawer of the incubator leads to an 89 dB level [38, 44, 49, 52].

The second loudest group of devices with a non-modifiable internal noise are respiratory devices, with High-Frequency Jet ventilators leading the way. The Jet patient box is encased in a plexiglass box to minimize the noise it produces, yet harmful high frequencies (up to 2000 Hz or pressure of 12 dB) are transmitted within the incubator [53]. Modern NICUs use a variety of respiratory modalities, all of which represent acoustic hazards. High-frequency oscillatory ventilator produces on average 60 dB intrinsic noise, with variation between 40 and 89. Conventional CPAP as well as bubble CPAP provide a range of 35–95 dB background noise, with an average of 55 dB [54]. That noise is delivered right to the oropharynx and has the potential to be transmitted directly to the middle ear. High-flow nasal cannula provides an average of 58 dB acoustic stimulation but can deliver up to 100 dB depending on the manufacturer and its flow [48, 54].

Eighteen percent of NICU graduates exposed to respiratory devices fail discharge hearing tests and 5% of those have persistent hearing loss on follow-up. Theories exist explaining why we do not see an even higher percentage of hearing loss despite prolonged exposure to noxious noise. One is that cartilage of the eustachian tune is quite soft in preterm neonates and is mostly found in a collapsed state, thus protecting the inner ear against direct noise transmission from the oropharynx to the middle ear [47–49, 55].

During in-hospital or inter-hospital transports noise levels can be very high. There are ways to reduce noise: reduce the sound from the source, block the sound, and protect the ear from the sound. Studies of disposable ear shells used in transport report reduction of 7–12 dB [54, 56]. Despite that, there is not enough evidence to recommend the routine use of such protectors during transport or in the NICU [40, 56]. Aminudin et al. [56], reported an increase in noise registered in the incubator during transport in babies who wore earmuffs [56]. Additionally, they demonstrated a 5–7% decrease in sound perception with active sound-canceling headphones, a promising technology that has not been widely developed for neonates [56].

5. NICU design

Environmental design research constitutes a distinct discipline that focuses on understanding the relationship between human interactions and the environment with a primary goal of improving the human condition and the well-being of individuals. In the context of the NICU, numerous studies have investigated the impact of architectural design and noise levels, proposing that the layout of the NICU plays a significant role in determining the amount of noise NICU patients and staffs are exposed to. Open bay rooms are characterized by having many patients sharing a single open area. Various sources contribute to a cacophony of noise in the open bay layout. These include essential life support equipment, heating, ventilation, and air conditioning (HVAC) systems, light buzzing, alarms triggered by vital sign monitoring devices, and the noise generated by staff conversation, occasional crying infants, and visiting family members. It is therefore reasonable to conclude that noise levels would be greater in this open environment. Research supports this observation. Open bay rooms were found to be louder than pods or private rooms and contributed to overall noise levels [2, 4, 5, 9].

The increased number of acoustic noise events in an open bay setup arises from the combined activities of patient care, visiting, conversations, and alarm activations [40, 51, 57]. In response to this issue, many modern NICU redesigns have increasingly adopted single or hybrid patient rooms equipped with sound-dampening technology [45]. In a 2018 study by Smith et al., the occurrence of peak sound levels exceeding 84 dB was found to be six times less frequent in private rooms when compared to the open room design [40]. Single-family rooms in the NICU have also demonstrated the potential to offer a more controlled and private environment, which may encourage parental presence and involvement in their infant's care and may even lead to a reduction in the length of stay [43].

While these design changes contributed to lower noise levels, some concerns have arisen. For instance, Pineda [43] highlighted that infants in quieter environments were exposed to seemingly less meaningful language, especially if they had fewer visitors and less parental engagement [43]. Meaningful language exposure was more evident when parents were present and engaged in their infant's care, more interactive, and held their infants more frequently [43].

Alternatively, a pod design, which consists of clustering four to six infants in adjoining rooms, may optimize infants' development and interaction with caregivers while potentially avoiding the isolation and reduction in meaningful language that can occur in private rooms lacking sufficient family engagement [58].

5.1 The effects of unwanted noise on staff

Studies have also evaluated how noisy NICUs and noise reduction strategies impact healthcare professionals. The findings indicate that staff experience significant stress as reported on the validated State-Trait Anxiety Inventory. They also report feelings of fatigue, difficulty concentrating, and tension headaches [17, 45]. Some staff shared that attempting to maintain a quiet environment and speak in low tones was a source of stress and seemed unrealistic especially when the NICU environment can become highly charged during crisis and acute situations [16].

6. NICU noise reduction interventions

Previous research suggests sound-reducing strategies for promoting a quiet NICU include environmental redesign, staff reminders, scheduled daily quiet time, ongoing education, silencing alarms quickly, and improved staffing ratios. In addition, sound levels are higher in Level III NICUs when compared to Level II NICUs, most likely related to the increased medical technologies utilized for the complex care required by Level III NICU patients. Due to the complex nature of a Level III NICU, more healthcare personnel are required giving rise to more HCP conversations, lifesaving interventions, alarms from cardiopulmonary instability, IV pumps, parent visitors, and general activity including environmental factors such as hospital-wide loudspeaker announcements, portable x-ray machines being wheeled into rooms, and recurrent, continuous, and sudden unexpected sounds, such as dropped objects or chairs being pulled across the floor [2–5].

Several intervention strategies have been evaluated, such as quiet time protocols, the use of visual noise feedback monitors, and staff "sound compliance supervisors" or a "peer-assisted" expert resource. These innovations were found to be effective in decreasing the level of noise during the study periods [5, 18–21]. In addition, Liszka et al. [24] and Zauche et al. [5] report that quiet time significantly decreased exposure to electronic sounds and voices concluding that a "quiet time" protocol could increase restful sleep and growth as well as foster a neuroprotective environment for at-risk neonates and may help improve cognition and language development in high-risk neonates [5, 24]. However, one study mentioned previously highlighted that infants in quieter environments were exposed to seemingly less meaningful language, especially if they had fewer visitors and less parental engagement [43].

Other strategies implemented included staff education programs, measuring sound levels, and infant position, or the application of earmuffs and eye shields in conjunction with measuring heart rate variability (HRV) or change in cerebral oxygenation during periods of elevated noise [1, 9, 18, 20, 21, 25–27, 59]. Elser et al. [25] and Gomes et al. [27] had conflicting results regarding the positive effect of positioning on the high-risk neonate's ability to reach physiologic stability in the presence of elevated noise [25, 27]. Aita et al. [26] looked at HRV and the use of earmuffs and eye shields and found no positive effect from this intervention. Although mixed results were discussed in these studies, it was again concluded that continued staff education and commitment are paramount to a sustained noise reduction program in the NICU [26].

On the horizon are technologies that include noise-canceling equipment. As mentioned earlier, one study examined the use of Bose Corporation QuietComfort 35 noise-canceling headphones on a neonatal mannequin housed within an isolette in an active NICU. Decibel levels were recorded at the mannequin ear level within the isolette and the noise level outside the isolette. It was found that 80% of the external SPL was detected at the mannequin ear with no protection. This was reduced by 5% with active noise-canceling, equivalent to approximately an 18 dB decrease (71 ± 4 dB decrease to 56 ± 1 dB) [56]. Another new technology is the prototype Active Noise Canceling Incubator which proposes to use Artificial Intelligence (AI) technology, and machine learning algorithms with feedback and feedforward to predict, analyze, and recreate an environment within the isolette to be as natural as possible for the NICU [60].

Batoca Silva et al. [52] surveyed health care professionals (HCP), including nurses, physicians, physiotherapists, and technical assistants, and reported that 77% of HCPs considered the NICU too noisy. Despite this perception, the results in our study show behaviors that seemed to demonstrate a lack of awareness of what they might be doing to decrease noise; for example, behaviors such as using a loud conventional voice at the bedside, failing to promptly silence alarms, and loudly opening and closing doors. Some HCPs may view their work environment as part of their personal space and not that of the sensitive environment of the developing preterm neonate [52].

Although the literature differs greatly in the forms of interventions and type of study design, the common themes in these studies support the evidence that noise in the NICU needs to be reduced. Future sound-reduction strategies should include adapting evidence to the local context, assessing barriers and facilitators to practice change, and including all HCPs and families in the planned design and implementation of interventions [51]. In addition, it is important to have a unit commitment to promote the growth and development of the neonate.

7. Authors' experience with a noise-reducing campaign

A pre- and post-observational study was conducted in a Level IV NICU in New York City. Interventions to reduce noise included: (1) novel approaches to multidisciplinary staff education program that included 22 disciplines involved in NICU care, including visual cues for when noise targets are exceeded, (2) parent education, including access to personal decibel meters, and (3) technical improvements to monitor alarm volume and electronic doors. Defined quiet ("HUSH") times were also instituted for 2 hours/shift. Educational and technical improvements were found to decrease median noise levels in the stepdown unit, but not in the acute care NICU. It was evident that the visual display failed to promote behaviors for noise reduction as noted in a study by Mayhew et al. [51]. In contrast, the HUSH program effectively reduced both noise and severe noise in both locations. Enforced focus on noise during the quiet times resulted in decreased noise levels throughout the day and night. Although there were limitations identified throughout this initiative, the HUSH strategy may be a sustainable way to decrease noise toxicity in the NICU to align with the American Academy of Pediatrics recommendations which remains a consistent observation as the literature available in addition to emphasizing staff education and a commitment to a "culture of silence."

8. Conclusion

Ample data supports the importance of developmentally appropriate noise exposure in utero and the NICU. Understanding the short-term pathologic sequelae as well as long-term growth and neurodevelopmental morbidities should encourage neonatal practitioners to monitor sound in the NICU. Ideally, as proposed by the US Environmental Protection Agency, a noise exceeding 45 dB will be avoided. Realistically, it is a very challenging task to implement consistently. Despite the challenge, units should implement quality improvement and education programs aiming to minimize exposure to high-frequency noise. Parental education on the importance of natural sounds must be provided and parent's presence, speech, and touch must be encouraged.

Medical practitioners should partner with industry to develop devices conducive to hearing protection, in addition to minimizing device-inherent noise generation. Modern NICU design should consider noise exposure as an important priority, influencing materials and construction surrounding our infants.

Based on our own experience, we believe that changing "the culture" of the unit is at the heart of sustainable change. Increasing staff awareness, providing education, instituting continuous audits, and "in real time" reminders can achieve consistently lower noise levels.

Author details

Vita Boyar[1,2]* and Annmarie Gennattasio[1,2]

1 Cohen Children's Medical Center of NY, Northwell Health, New Hyde Park, NY, USA

2 Donald and Barbara Zucker School of Medicine at Hofstra, Northwell, USA

*Address all correspondence to: vboyar@gmail.com

References

[1] Calikusu, Incekar M, Balci S. The effect of training on noise reduction in neonatal intensive care units. Journal for Specialists in Pediatric Nursing. 2017;**22**(3):e12181

[2] Capriolo C, Viscardi RM, Broderick KA, Nassebeh S, Kochan M, Solanki NS, et al. Assessment of neonatal intensive care unit sound exposure using a smartphone application. American Journal of Perinatology. Jan 2022;**39**(2):189-194

[3] Casavant SG, Bernier K, Andrews S, Bourgoin A. Noise in the neonatal intensive care unit: What does the evidence tell us? Advances in Neonatal Care: Official Journal of the National Association of Neonatal Nurses. 2017;**17**(4):265-273

[4] Hernández-Salazar AD, Gallegos-Martínez J, Reyes-Hernández J. Level and noise sources in the neonatal intensive care unit of a reference hospital. Investigación y Educación en Enfermería. 2020;**38**(3):e13

[5] Zauche LH, Zauche MS, Williams BL. Influence of quiet time on the auditory environment of infants in the NICU. JOGNN-Journal of Obstetric, Gynecologic, & Neonatal Nursing. 2021;**50**(1):68-77

[6] Almadhoob A, Ohlsson A. Sound reduction management in the neonatal intensive care unit for preterm or very low birth weight infants. Cochrane Database of Systematic Reviews. 2020;**1**:CD010333

[7] Goines L, Hagler L. Noise pollution: A modem plague. Southern Medical Journal. 2007;**100**(3):287-294

[8] Hill JN, LaVela SL. Noise levels in patient rooms and at nursing stations at three VA medical centers. HERD. 2015;**9**(1):54-63

[9] Hu L, Liu Q, Yuan H, Lu C, Zhou W. Efficacy of noise reduction bundle in reducing sound levels in a level II neonatal care unit in China. Translational Pediatrics. 2020;**9**(6):750-756

[10] Rhee CJ, da Costa CS, Austin T, Brady KM, Czosnyka M, Lee JK. Neonatal cerebrovascular autoregulation. Pediatric Research. 2018;**84**(5):602-610

[11] Vesoulis ZA, Mathur AM. Cerebral autoregulation, brain injury, and the transitioning premature infant. Frontiers in Pediatrics. 2017;**5**:64

[12] Robinson S. Neonatal posthemorrhagic hydrocephalus from prematurity: Pathophysiology and current treatment concepts. Journal of Neurosurgery: Pediatrics [Internet]. 2012;**9**(3). Available from: https://www.ncbi.nlm.nih.gov/pmc/articles/PMC3842211/ [cited: April 1, 2021]

[13] Larson L. Can you hear me now? Kentucky Nurse. 2010;**58**(3):10

[14] Singh M, Parvez B, Banquet A, Kase JS. Habilitation of very preterm infants at a Post Acute Care Inpatient Rehabilitation (PACIR) center after neonatal intensive care unit (NICU) discharge. Developmental Neurorehabilitation. 2019;**22**(1):53-60

[15] Khajenasiri F, Zamanian A, Zamanian Z. The effect of exposure to high noise levels on the performance and rate of error in manual activities. Electronic Physician. 2016;**8**(3):2088-2093

[16] Swathi S, Ramesh A, Nagapoornima M, Fernandes LM,

Jisina C, Rao PNS, et al. Sustaining a "culture of silence" in the neonatal intensive care unit during nonemergency situations: A grounded theory on ensuring adherence to behavioral modification to reduce noise levels. International Journal of Qualitative Studies on Health and Well-Being. 2014;**9**:22523

[17] Terzi B, Azizoğlu F, Polat Ş, Kaya N, İşsever H. The effects of noise levels on nurses in intensive care units. Nursing in Critical Care. 2019;**24**(5):299-305

[18] Casey L, Fucile S, Flavin M, Dow K. A two-pronged approach to reduce noise levels in the neonatal intensive care unit. Early Human Development. 2020;**146**:105073

[19] Pugliesi RR, Campillos MS, Calado Orsi KCS, Avena MJ, de Cacia Pradella-Hallinan ML, Tsunemi MH, et al. Correlation of premature infant sleep/wakefulness and noise levels in the presence or absence of "quiet time". Advances in Neonatal Care: Official Journal of the National Association of Neonatal Nurses. 2018;**18**(5):393-399

[20] Wang D, Aubertin C, Barrowman N, Moreau K, Dunn S, Harrold J. Reduction of noise in the neonatal intensive care unit using sound-activated noise meters. Archives of Disease in Childhood. Fetal and Neonatal Edition. 2014;**99**(6):F515-F516

[21] Biabanakigoortani A, Namnabati M, Abdeyazdan Z, Badii Z. Effect of peer education on the noise management in Iranian neonatal intensive care unit. Iranian Journal of Nursing and Midwifery Research. 2016;**21**(3):317-321

[22] Craig JW, Glick C, Phillips R, Hall SL, Smith J, Browne J. Recommendations for involving the family in developmental care of the NICU baby. Journal of Perinatology. 2015;**35**(1):S5-S8

[23] Pineda R, Bender J, Hall B, Shabosky L, Annecca A, Smith J. Parent participation in the neonatal intensive care unit: Predictors and relationships to neurobehavior and developmental outcomes. Early Human Development. 2018;**117**:32-38

[24] Liszka L, Smith J, Mathur A, Schlaggar BL, Colditz G, Pineda R. Differences in early auditory exposure across neonatal environments. Early Human Development. 2019;**136**:27-32

[25] Elser HE, Holditch-Davis D, Levy J, Brandon DH. The effects of environmental noise and infant position on cerebral oxygenation. Advances in Neonatal Care: Official Journal of the National Association of Neonatal Nurses. 2012;**12**(Suppl. 5):S18-S27

[26] Aita M, Johnston C, Goulet C, Oberlander TF, Snider L. Intervention minimizing preterm infants' exposure to NICU light and noise. Clinical Nursing Research. 2013;**22**(3):337-358

[27] de Freitas Dantas Gomes EL, Santos CMD, da Costa Souza Santos A, da Silva AG, França MAM, Romanini DS, et al. Autonomic responses of premature newborns to body position and environmental noise in the neonatal intensive care unit. Revista Brasileira de Terapia Intensiva. 2019;**31**(3):296-302

[28] Darcy AE, Hancock LE, Ware EJ. A descriptive study of noise in the neonatal intensive care unit. Ambient levels and perceptions of contributing factors. Advances in Neonatal Care: Official Journal of the National Association of Neonatal Nurses. 2008;**8**(3):165-175

[29] The Lancet Regional Health–Europe. Noise pollution: More attention is needed. The Lancet Regional Health-Europe. 2023;**24**:100577

[30] Utzong. Types of Noise-SoundEar Int. Believes in Creating Awareness About Noise [Internet]. SoundEar Int.; 2021. Available from: https://soundear.com/types-of-noise/ [cited: September 17, 2023]

[31] Farooqi ZUR, Ahmad I, Ditta A, Ilic P, Amin M, Naveed AB, et al. Types, sources, socioeconomic impacts, and control strategies of environmental noise: A review. Environmental Science and Pollution Research International. 2022;**29**(54):81087-81111

[32] Sloan M. Noise Colors: Which One Is Best for Sleep? Discover Magazine; 2023. Available from: https://www.discovermagazine.com/health/noise-colors-which-one-is-best-for-sleep [cited: September 17, 2023]

[33] Definition of HERTZ [Internet]. 2023. Available from: https://www.merriam-webster.com/dictionary/hertz [cited: September 17, 2023]

[34] Definition of Brownian Motion [Internet]. Available from: https://www.merriam-webster.com/dictionary/Brownian+motion [cited: September 17, 2023]

[35] Manhattan Neighborhood Network [Internet]. The Basics of Sound: What Are Frequency and Amplitude? 2022. Available from: https://www.mnn.org/blog/basics-sound-what-are-frequency-and-amplitude [cited: September 17, 2023]

[36] How Is Sound Measured? Noisy Planet [Internet]; 2019. Available from: https://www.noisyplanet.nidcd.nih.gov/have-you-heard/how-is-sound-measured [cited: September 17, 2023]

[37] Sound Pressure Level (SPL) and the Decibel Scale (dB) 101 [Internet]. 2019. Available from: https://www.youtube.com/watch?v=8q-6jqh2Qdc [cited: September 17, 2023]

[38] Reuter C, Bartha-Doering L, Czedik-Eysenberg I, Maeder M, Bertsch M, Bibl K, et al. Living in a box: Understanding acoustic parameters in the NICU environment-PMC. Frontiers in Pediatrics [Internet]. 2023. Available from: https://www-ncbi-nlm-nih-gov.medproxy.hofstra.edu/pmc/articles/PMC10083238/ [cited: September 13, 2023]

[39] Lahav A, Skoe E. An acoustic gap between the NICU and womb: A potential risk for compromised neuroplasticity of the auditory system in preterm infants. Frontiers in Neuroscience. 2014;**8**:381

[40] Smith SW, Ortmann AJ, Clark WW. Noise in the neonatal intensive care unit: A new approach to examining acoustic events. Noise & Health. 2018;**20**(95):121-130

[41] Noise: A hazard for the fetus and newborn. American Academy of Pediatrics. Committee on Environmental Health. Pediatrics. 1997;**100**(4):724-727

[42] McMahon E, Wintermark P, Lahav A. Auditory brain development in premature infants: The importance of early experience. Annals of the New York Academy of Sciences. 2012;**1252**(1):17-24

[43] Pineda R, Durant P, Mathur A, Inder T, Wallendorf M, Schlaggar BL. Auditory exposure in the neonatal intensive care unit: Room type and other predictors. The Journal of Pediatrics. 2017;**183**:56-66.e3

[44] Monson BB, Rock J, Cull M, Soloveychik V. Neonatal intensive care unit incubators reduce language and noise levels more than the womb. Journal of Perinatology: Official Journal of

the California Perinatal Association. 2020;**40**(4):600-606

[45] Verderber S, Gray S, Suresh-Kumar S, Kercz D, Parshuram C. Intensive care unit built environments: A comprehensive literature review (2005-2020). Health Environments Research and Design Journal. 2021;**14**(4):368-415

[46] Miller RW, Brendel WB, Brent RL, Chisolm JJ, Doyle JL, Ebbin AJ, et al. Noise pollution: Neonatal aspects. Pediatrics. 1974;**54**(4):476-479

[47] Williams AL, Sanderson M, Lai D, Selwyn BJ, Lasky RE. Intensive care noise and mean arterial blood pressure in extremely low-birth-weight neonates. American Journal of Perinatology. 2009;**26**(5):323-329

[48] Wachman EM, Lahav A. The effects of noise on preterm infants in the NICU. Archives of Disease in Childhood. Fetal and Neonatal Edition. 2011;**96**(4):F305-F309

[49] Bertsch M, Reuter C, Czedik-Eysenberg I, Berger A, Olischar M, Bartha-Doering L, et al. The "sound of silence" in a neonatal intensive care unit—listening to speech and music inside an incubator. Frontiers in Psychology [Internet]. 2020;**11**. Available from: https://www.frontiersin.org/article/10.3389/fpsyg.2020.01055 [cited: May 19, 2022]

[50] Carvalhais C, Da Silva MV, Xavier A, Santos J. Good practices to reduce noise levels in the neonatal intensive care unit. In: Arezes PM, Baptista JS, Barroso MP, Carneiro P, Cordeiro P, Costa N, et al., editors. Occupational and Environmental Safety and Health [Internet]. Cham: Springer International Publishing; 2019. pp. 297-302. (Studies in Systems, Decision and Control; Vol. 202). Available from: http://link.springer.com/10.1007/978-3-030-14730-3_32 [cited: September 13, 2023]

[51] Mayhew KJ, Lawrence SL, Squires JE, Harrison D. Elevated sound levels in the neonatal intensive care unit: What is causing the problem? Advances in Neonatal Care: Official Journal of the National Association of Neonatal Nurses. 2022;**22**(6):E207-E216

[52] Batoca Silva EM, Ramos A, Duarte J, Marques da Silva D. Noise in neonatology: Perception of health professionals. Revista de Enfermagem Referencia. 2019;**IV Série**:67-76

[53] Marik PE, Fuller C, Levitov A, Moll E. Neonatal incubators: A toxic sound environment for the preterm infant?*. Pediatric Critical Care Medicine. 2012;**13**(6):685-689

[54] Singh D, Fusch G. Investigating noise exposure to newborn infants from respiratory support: Methodological considerations. Cureus. 2021;**13**(11):e19353

[55] Massa-Buck B, Rastogi D, Rastogi S. Complications associated with incorrect use of nasal CPAP. Journal of Perinatology: Official Journal of the California Perinatal Association. 2023 Aug;**43**(8):975-981

[56] Aminudin N, Franta J, Bowden A, Corcoran JD, El-Khuffash A, McCallion N. Noise exposure exceeded safe limits during neonatal care and road transport but was reduced by active noise cancelling. Acta Paediatrica (Oslo, Norway : 1992). 1992;**112**(10):2060-2065

[57] Parra J, de Suremain A, Berne Audeoud F, Ego A, Debillon T. Sound levels in a neonatal intensive care unit significantly exceeded recommendations, especially inside incubators. Acta

Paediatrica (Oslo, Norway: 1992). 2017;**106**(12):1909-1914

[58] Aita M, Robins S, Charbonneau L, Doray-Demers P, Feeley N. Comparing light and noise levels before and after a NICU change of design. Journal of Perinatology: Official Journal of the California Perinatal Association. 2021;**41**(9):2235-2243

[59] Jousselme C, Vialet R, Jouve E, Lagier P, Martin C, Michel F. Efficacy and mode of action of a noise-sensor light alarm to decrease noise in the pediatric intensive care unit: A prospective, randomized study*. Pediatric Critical Care Medicine. 2011;**12**(2):e69-e72

[60] Jaschke AC, Bos AF. Concept and considerations of a medical device: The active noise cancelling incubator. Frontiers in Pediatrics. 2023;**11**:1187815

Chapter 6

Phototherapy: Safe and Effective Use of Light in Neonatal Care

Janet Carvajal de la Osa, Yenisel Díaz Roller and Iosvany Aguiar Ramos

Abstract

Light is a very effective tool for the treatment of neonates with problems at birth. It includes different wavelengths that can cause damage for different reasons when misused. Taking into account the characteristics of the light rays applied to neonates is important in the field of phototherapy, for the application of good clinical practices and prudent avoidance, in risk management. In this chapter, research on the application of phototherapy will be presented, highlighting the non-visible risks of using light in incubators and thermal cradles. In addition, recommendations will be made about specific aspects regarding the use and application of light for both neonate. The results show that the application of phototherapy increases the levels of electromagnetic radiation. Therefore, it must be taken into account that, although it is of vital importance for the care of preterm neonates, artificial light is a tool whose operation depends on electrical energy and represents a risk that could subsequently affect their state of health.

Keywords: electromagnetic field, light spectrum, phototherapy, preterm neonate, photonic radiation

1. Introduction

Jaundice is the yellowish discoloration of the skin and mucous membranes caused by the accumulation or deposit of bilirubin, which, according to clinical data, occurs in 60–70% of newborns [1]. Some authors claim that in newborns (NB), it is a condition that can cause neuronal damage when there are excessive amounts of it, producing permanent neurological sequelae in the patient [2]. This is why this pathological condition must be prevented by maintaining safe levels of bilirubin in the blood. To achieve these levels, phototherapy has been one of the most used techniques, through which the transformation of bilirubin into water-soluble photoisomers is achieved thanks to the effect of light on it, which allows them to be more easily excreted through feces and urine, without the need to be conjugated in the liver [3].

Phototherapy is a technique used in neonates to combat certain conditions that occur in them during birth, high levels of bilirubin being one of them. These phototherapy units are made up of four blue light tubes and two white light tubes. The blue ones are placed in the center, and the white ones on the sides. Light tubes or bulbs, whether LED, halogen, or fluorescent, are classified according to the maximum wavelength produced by the emitted light. Among the different types, there are: specialized blue fluorescent lamps, compact fluorescent lamps and halogen spotlights or lamps with an LED system. Some of these are also used to illuminate the work area in general.

Fluorescent tubes have plexiglass shields to filter out any ultraviolet radiation and do not emit dangerous levels of infrared radiation. LED bulbs emit blue light that does not increase temperature or emit ultraviolet radiation. However, these bulbs, with high levels of radiation, can damage the eyes and skin, so they must include internal filters and reflectors to reduce them.

2. Light characteristics

According to Maxwell's theory [4], light is a wavelength perturbation in an electromagnetic field in the form of radiation that propagates at a defined speed. Their characteristics are:

- Amplitude (wave height).
- Wavelength (spatial behavior): λ (nm).
- Speed: c (km/sec) is the distance the wave travels in 1 second.
- Frequency (temporal behavior): v (hz), defined by the number of waves that pass a fixed point in one second. It is related to the wavelength, since it depends on its size. It is estimated at the wavelength multiplied by 1014 cycles per second.

Light is transmitted in a vacuum at the speed of 299,792.458 km/sec, according to Einstein's theory of relativity, comprising different wavelengths and frequencies. When the medium changes, its speed and wavelength change, but its frequency remains constant [5], as shown in **Figure 1**.

The electromagnetic spectrum is nothing more than the arrangement of radiant energy according to wavelength (λ) or frequency. It extends from wavelengths of 10^{16} to 10^{-7} m, as seen in **Figure 2**. At the lower end are the highest frequencies, which

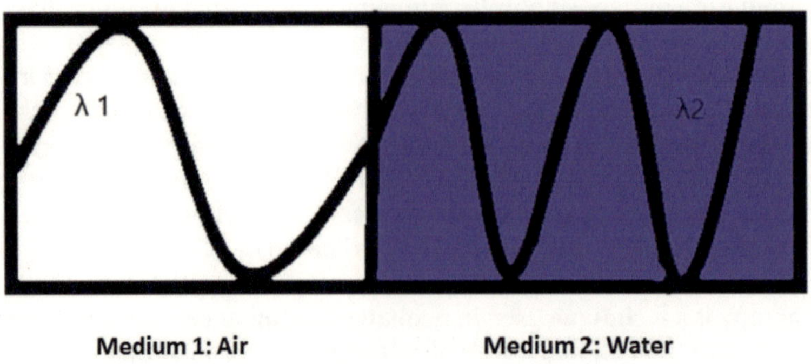

Figure 1.
Behavior of light from one medium to another. [own creation].

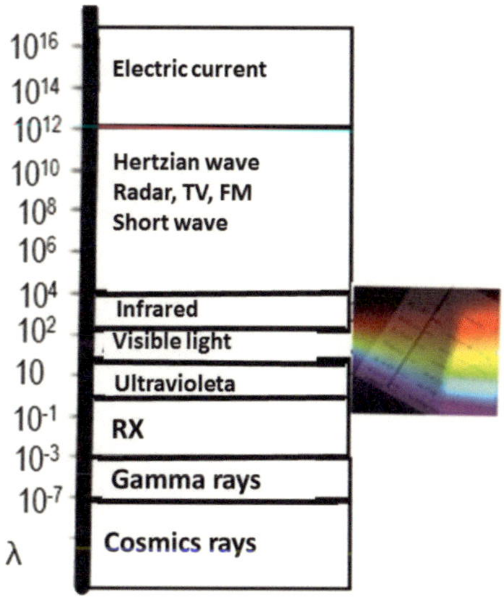

Figure 2.
Electromagnetic spectrum. [own creation].

are the short wave and the highest energy, equivalent to cosmic rays. On the opposite side, long waves can be found, whose wavelength is highly variable and are used for radio communications, where X-ray, ultraviolet (UV), visible, and infrared (IR) rays are located.

It can be said that the three major regions of importance in the field of lighting are infrared light, visible light, and ultraviolet light. However, despite being so significant for human life, the visible spectrum corresponds to a tiny portion of the spectrum of electromagnetic waves. Although UV and IR rays are not detected by the human eye, their effect can be noticed physiologically. To measure the visible spectrum, the most used unit of measurement is the nanometer (nm), which is equivalent to 10^{-9} m.

2.1 Light spectrum

The light spectrum is nothing more than the decomposition of white or visible light into colors that delimit its wavelengths [6]. This ranges from ultraviolet to infrared, defined between wavelengths that range approximately from 380 to 770 nm, as can be seen in **Figure 3**.

Perceived white light, as mentioned above, is a mixture of all visible wavelengths. The visible spectrum can be broken down into its different wavelengths using a quartz prism, which refracts each of them selectively through colors. The human eye separates, by capturing color, each of the different wavelengths and frequencies present in this range.

Each wavelength interval is represented by a color:

- Blue and violet correspond to short wavelengths, approximately 380 to 500 nm.
- Red and orange correspond to long wavelengths, approximately 590 to 700 nm.
- Green and yellow are found in the middle zone, which covers wavelengths from 500 to 590 nm.

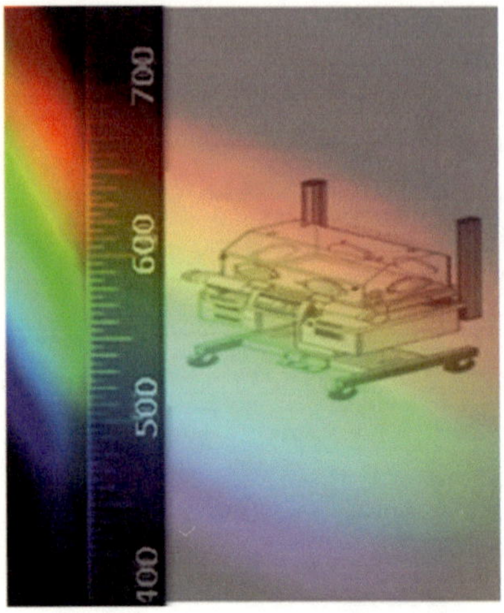

Figure 3.
Light spectrum. [own creation].

Achieving monochromatic light radiation, that is, one that responds to a single wavelength, is very difficult. The light sources that most closely resemble this type of emission are the laser and the low-pressure sodium lamp.

Radiant energy is made up of electromagnetic waves with a range of frequencies (v) ranging from 108 to 1024 s^{-1} and propagates at a constant speed (of light), whose value is exactly 299,792,458 m/s [5].

2.1.1 White light

White light is the result of the sum of countless wavelengths that, when added, become colored rays, giving rise to the perception of the color white. As stated by Mosquera Torres et al. [7], white light is 25% blue light.

Most lamps intended for lighting work areas in the health sector emit white light. This condition is necessary for the safety and protection of management and the health of both patients and workers.

2.1.2 Blue light

Basically, phototherapy applied to neonates with conditions at birth is based on the use of blue and white light. Wavelengths between 380 and 500 nm include the violet, blue, and green areas of the spectrum [8]. This part of the spectrum is also known as high-energy, short-wavelength visible light.

Sunlight is the main natural source of blue light, although there are enough sources of artificial blue light for humans to be exposed 24 hours a day. In 2013, a panel of American experts [8] pointed out that solar radiation is 25–30% blue light, as shown in the spectrum in **Figure 4**.

All artificial light sources have blue light in their spectrum in different percentages; thus, conventional incandescent light lamps have the least with around 3%, low consumption compact fluorescent lamps at approximately 26%, and LED lamps, which emit cool white light, blue light is 35% one of the strongest components [8], as shown in **Figure 5**.

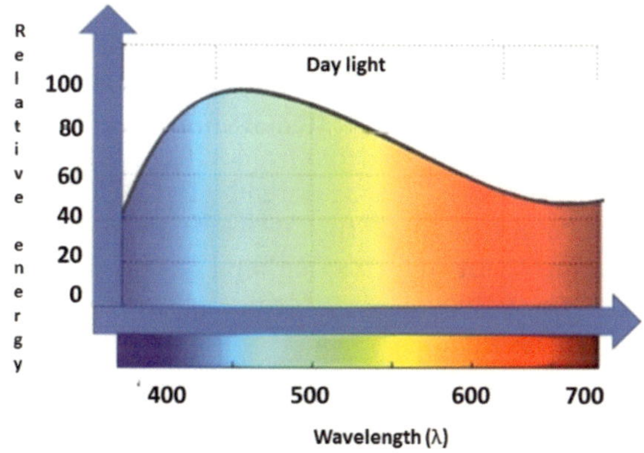

Figure 4.
Representation of the daylight spectrum. [own creation].

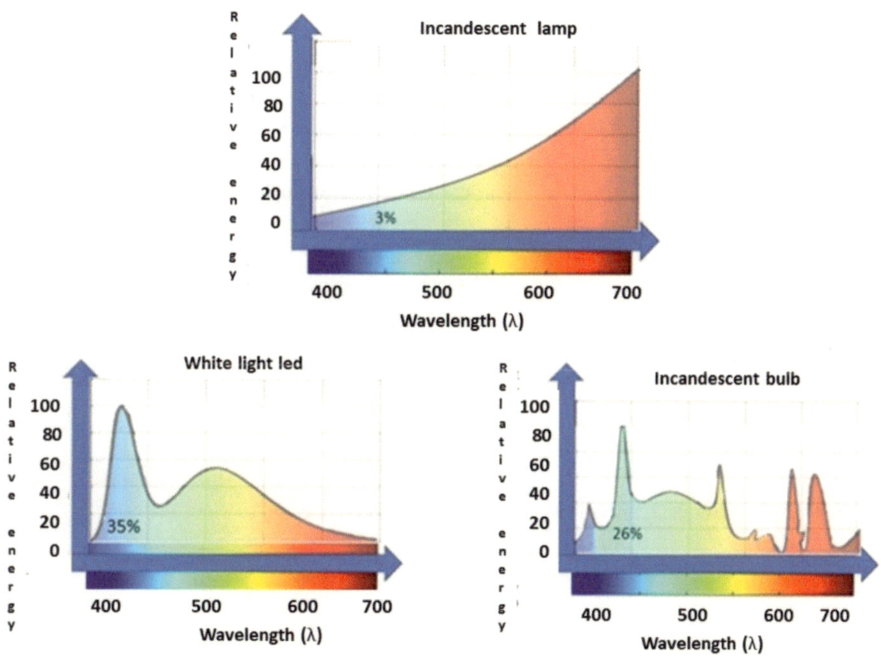

Figure 5.
Representation of the spectrum of some artificial light sources. [own creation].

Jiménez-Rubio et al. [9] mention that blue light provides benefits to the synchronization of circadian cycles and the production of melatonin, if it is properly provided during the day and night cycles, also as it has been shown to provide the newborn with high levels of bilirubin an effective treatment [10], but at the same time, it must be taken into account that the indiscriminate use of this type of light poses specific risks to vision and skin that are irreversible due to its power of penetration into biological material [11].

For their part, studies carried out in the last decade have suggested that phototherapy is associated with type 1 diabetes [12, 13], damage to the immune system, leukemias [14], and asthma [15] as late and long-term effects. The relationship, according to these investigations, is due to the fact that by applying phototherapy 24 hours a day, the neonate is inhibited from producing what is necessary to raise the immature immune level. This situation, as stated by Boidi [16], causes a deficiency of T lymphocytes, molecular alterations in the DNA of mononuclear leukocytes, alterations in the concentrations of interleukins that tend to slow down the change in an immune response, increasing the risk of suffering in the long term—the mentioned diseases.

3. Lighting environment in a neonatal intensive care unit

Currently, there are no standards that standardize adequate light levels in a Neonatal Intensive Care Unit (NICU), as this structurally depends on the geographical characteristics of the place, the type of care provided in the unit, and the design and location of the Windows. Additionally, the condition of the newborn and its location within the area must be taken into account.

For premature babies, reducing light, as well as maintaining the light and dark cycle, is of vital importance, which is why it is convenient to have intensity regulators to adjust the light power depending on the needs that arise daily around them. Him.

As recommendations to maintain the minimum lighting conditions, it is adopted that, during the day, the light oscillates between 100 and 200 lux, preferably supported by natural light and, at night, artificial light of approximately 50 lux, but allowing it to be adapted between 10 and 600 lux independently depending on the case [17]. If a short-term evaluation of a specific RN is necessary, between 1000 and 1500 lux can be used, avoiding interference with nearby children.

In nursing work areas, it is advisable to have moderate levels of lighting with the possibility of regulation and during the day to take advantage of natural light, somewhat distorting its direct action on the work area.

3.1 Types of phototherapy that an incubator can offer

Today, there are several modalities of phototherapy such as:

- White light, which is used everywhere (in the thermal crib (TC) or radiant crib, in the case of premature babies).

- Blue light and fiber optic or biwhite light (in which the child can be dressed during phototherapy and phototherapy can be performed at home).

- High-intensity phototherapies, which are double phototherapies, have shown greater benefits.

The effectiveness of phototherapy depends on the irradiation of the light source. Irradiance is expressed in units of watts or microwatts per square centimeter per nanometer ($W/cm^2/nm$) ($\mu W/cm^2/nm$), respectively, within a given wavelength band [3].

Depending on the maximum wavelength produced by light and the hours of exposure to it, there are different types of phototherapy, such as:

1. Simple, standard, or conventional phototherapy: radiation of 8–10 μW/cm^2/nm emitted by a lamp with fluorescent tubes, two white and four blue, is used.

2. Intermittent or continuous phototherapy: as the name indicates, it works with cycles of light exposure and cycles of rest. The lamps used for standard phototherapy are used and are classified as:

   - Intermittent phototherapy: characterized by cycles of light exposure and rest cycles, it is normally composed of 12 hours of exposure and 12 hours of rest. Only simple or conventional phototherapy can be applied intermittently.

   - Continuous phototherapy: in this type of phototherapy, light exposure is carried out 24 hours a day, pausing only during essential moments such as feeding or diaper changes.

3. Double or intensive phototherapy: uses radiation greater than 30 μW/cm^2/nm and uses lamps with six blue tubes.

Miriam Janet de la Rosa [18] suggests that, when placed 20 cm above the newborn, phototherapy units with conventional or standard light should provide spectral irradiation of 8–10 μW/cm^2/nm, in the 430–490 nm, while special blue fluorescent lamps provide 30–40 μW/cm^2/nm, in that same band.

On the other hand, there are investigations [1, 19] that show that the benefits that light therapy provides on bilirubin have reported negative clinical results on the pathophysiology of NBs, such as lower weight gain, alterations in sleep development and stress in very premature or seriously ill patients. What could be associated with electromagnetic radiation resulting from the use of electrical energy to keep the phototherapy equipment and other elements that make up preterm NB treatments in operation?

4. Electromagnetic fields

Electromagnetic fields (EMF) are a combination of electrical and magnetic waves that travel simultaneously [20]. They propagate at the speed of light and are characterized by a frequency and its corresponding wavelength. These two characteristics are directly related to each other: the higher the frequency, the shorter the wavelength. All equipment that needs to be connected to the electrical energy network emits electromagnetic radiation when it comes into operation. Light lamps of all types have this condition, which is why they emit electromagnetic radiation.

According to the Council of the European Union, the basic constraint limit allowed for any point or spatial measurement is equivalent to a magnetic induction (β) of 6.25 μT [21]. Electromagnetic radiation capable of exciting the retina and creating the sensation of vision belongs to the area of the spectrum called visible light, as shown in **Figure 2**.

Electromagnetic radiation has been recognized by the World Health Organization (WHO) since 2002 [22] to cause health damage. This damage is subject to the behavior of different variables, such as:

- Exhibition time
- Radiation level
- Distance at which the source of the radiation object is located
- Person's health criterion
- Adding fields near the radiation source.

Electromagnetic fields are not subtracted; they only add the radiation that they emanate to others and themselves. To reduce the levels of radiation that reach the irradiated object, it must be taken into account at what distance to place it. Issue that is regulated by the International Electrotechnical Commission (IEC) to avoid interference between equipment. In the case of lamps or luminaires, it is recommended that they be located approximately 1.5 m away from people, due to the levels of radiation they emit.

5. Demonstrating theories

The objective of this research is to demonstrate that the use of light in intensive care units brings dangers that are not taken into account by the people dedicated to working in them, either because it is not visible or due to a lack of knowledge.

For this, a research protocol divided into three stages was drawn up:

Stage 1: The magnetic field of the NICU area was measured using a PCE-G28 gaussmeter. This area includes a monitoring cubicle (indicated as 1) and seven confinement cubicles for the care of neonates (indicated from 2 to 8).

- The gaussmeter was placed one meter away from the ground (the height at which the babies are lying), meter by meter was measured in a timely manner, moving the measuring equipment throughout the area and always starting with the area furthest from the entrance door and counterclockwise.

Stage 2: The magnetic field radiated by an incubator with only six months of operation and a thermal cradle with the same operating time was measured. The measurements were carried out in isolated rooms where no medical equipment coexisted around them and turned on one at a time. Furthermore, these values were taken with the incorporation of light therapy, to use them as a behavioral pattern of emitted radiation for future comparisons.

- The gaussmeter was positioned vertically on the four sides of the incubators and thermal cradles, averaging the specific value to which the baby would be subjected while inside it. This operation was performed five times to achieve statistical validation.
- For this, the percentage, chosen by brand and model, that these would occupy within the equipment in operation, at the time of the investigation, was taken into account.

Stage 3: The values irradiated by the incubators and thermal cradles were measured during their operation in each of the cubicles in the area to be investigated, using the same procedure as for the reference standard. A comparison graph was made with respect to the pattern measured in isolation, taking into account those that were applying light and those that were not.

Note: The investigation was carried out with a general air conditioning regime and light on only in the measured areas.

As a result of the application of the methodology explained above, the color maps shown below were obtained; these represent the magnetic field values irradiated in each of the stages mentioned above. For greater understanding, they will be presented in stages.

5.1 Stage 1

In this stage, general magnetic field values were obtained in each cubicle. They are represented by a color map in **Figure 6**.

The color bar shows that the highest radiation values are above 2 μT, represented in yellow, and can be observed in specific areas that symbolize the presence of a magnetic field generator in operation. The generators in this case are incubators and thermal cradles with or without phototherapy light applied.

5.2 Stage 2

For this stage of the research, the percentage of incubators in terms of brand and model was taken into account, and the one with the shortest operating time was taken, in the same way as thermal cribs. The values obtained from the measurements are presented, as averaged in **Table 1**.

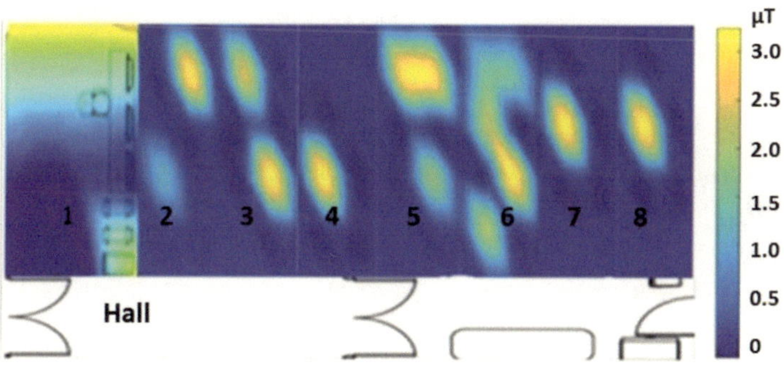

Figure 6.
Color map of the magnetic field of the general area with the equipment in operation.

Equipment	Average of five measurements	
	Light off	Light on
ATOM Medical V-85 Incubator	0.68 μT	1.17 μT
Medix Thermal Crib	0.45 μT	0.93 μT

Table 1.
Measurements were made in an incubator and a thermal cradle to obtain a behavior pattern with respect to magnetic field radiation.

With respect to technological equipment, ten incubators were in use, eight of which were Atom Medical V-85 brand (located in cubicles 2, 3, 4, 5, 7, and 8) and five thermal cribs, all of which were Medix brand. (located in cubicle 6). All equipment in operation has been in that condition for more than five years.

5.3 Stage 3

Once the reference values to be used were obtained, the magnetic fields irradiated by the equipment in operation were measured following the protocol of stage 2. The values grouped in **Table 2** were obtained. The light used was continuous blue light.

As has been proven by some researchers, as electrical or electronic equipment comes into operation, the ambient magnetic field of the area increases its radiation level.

In **Figure 7**, the range of colors shows the difference in the levels of electromagnetic radiation radiated by the incubators. In this figure, it can be seen that:

- In cubicle 2, incubator 1 has an intense yellow color that indicates a higher level of radiation (2.30 μT), while in incubator 2 it has a blue color that, according to the color bar, represents lower levels (0.66 μT, in this case).

- In cubicle 5, the difference is revealed between incubator 3 and incubators 1 and 2 (approximately from 2.0 to 2.47 μT), showing that as the blue light treatment of phototherapy is incorporated, they reach higher values in incubators 1 and 2 (2.20 and 2.67 μT, respectively), than the value obtained in incubator 3 (0.2 μT), which does not have associated phototherapy.

Cubicle	Equipment	Light on	Light off	Reference
2	Incubator 1	2.30 μT		1.17 μT
	Incubator 2		0.66 μT	0.68 μT
3	Incubator 1	2.22 μT		1.17 μT
	Incubator 2	1.87 μT		
4	Incubator 1	2.15 μT		
5	Incubator 1	2.20 μT		
	Incubator 2	2.67 μT		
	Incubator 3		0.2 μT	0.68 μT
6	Thermal crib 4		0.84 μT	0.45 μT
	Thermal crib 5		0.5 μT	
	Thermal crib 6		0.54 μT	
	Thermal crib 7		0.45 μT	
	Thermal crib 8	2.1 μT		0.93 μT
7	Incubator 1	2.19 μT		1.17 μT
8	Incubator 1	2.19 μT		

Table 2.
Table showing the magnetic field radiated by the equipment in operation, at the time of measurement with the phototherapy light on or off.

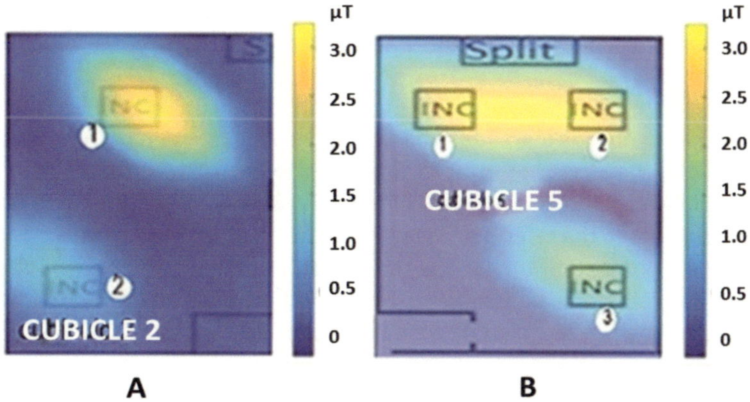

Figure 7.
Representation of the difference in electromagnetic radiation generated by incubators with phototherapy, (A) 1 and (B) 1 and 2 and without phototherapy included in the treatment of preterm newborns, (A) 2 and (B) 3.

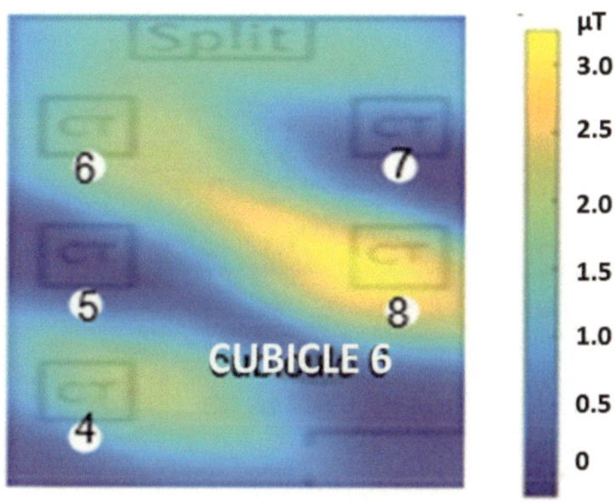

Figure 8.
Representation of the difference in electromagnetic irradiation, through colors, while the phototherapy treatment is applied in the thermal cots in cubicle 6.

The difference in values represented between (A) and (B) for the incubators where the use of phototherapy is present, could be given by the exploitation time, an issue that influences one of the factors mentioned above as a behavioral variable of the electromagnetic field. Also, the amount of equipment used in the treatment to keep the newborn alive is sometimes between 4 and 5, located around the incubator.

Figure 8 represents the behavior of electromagnetic radiation, when the phototherapy lights are working or not. During the operation of the thermal cradles, it is represented by the display of colors whose values are incorporated numerically in the bar. In the thermal cribs located in cubicle 6, only five cribs were providing service, and the only one that had the phototherapy treatment incorporated was number 8 (2.1 μT), and this is expressed by the intense yellow color that is represented in the map. Here, it can be seen that the difference between values when phototherapy is being applied and, when not, ranges approximately between 1.2 and 2 μT, values lower than the difference shown in the comparison of the incubators.

If the reference patterns are taken into account with respect to the values measured during the investigation, to make a comparison about the levels reached by this life support equipment in a NICU, the graphs shown in **Figures 9** and **10** were obtained. They will be shown separately depending on whether the equipment incorporates light therapy or not.

If the values obtained for electromagnetic radiation are compared with respect to the reference standards (Inc. Ref. and CT Ref.), it can be seen in the graphs of **Figures 9** and **10** that, except for incubator 2 of cubicle 2 (Inc. 2 cub. 2) and incubator 3 of cubicle 5 (Inc. 3 cub. 5), which do not have incorporated light treatment, the rest have values above the reference. This issue can be attributed to the presence in its surroundings of other equipment used in the treatment of the baby. This shows that electromagnetic radiation, being invisible, is not taken into account for diagnostic treatment in incubators and the application of phototherapy treatment.

Incubators and thermal cribs are quintessential equipment for exclusive use in NICUs. It is known that they provide the preterm newborn with comfort and safety, but incubators are electrical equipment that provide electromagnetic fields and this, in turn, exerts influences on body parameters responsible for maintaining the physiological safety of the newborn.

When using phototherapy on a baby who is in an incubator, you are providing photonic radiation, which emits a level of electromagnetic radiation that, in turn, is

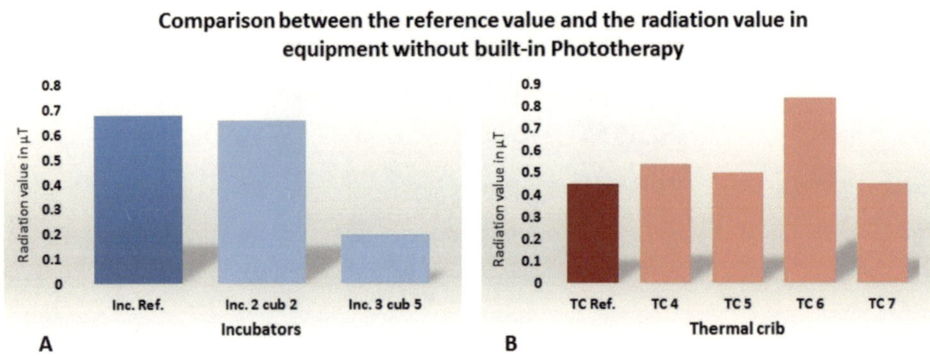

Figure 9.
Comparison graphs of electromagnetic radiation without applying phototherapy in incubator (A) and thermal cradles (B).

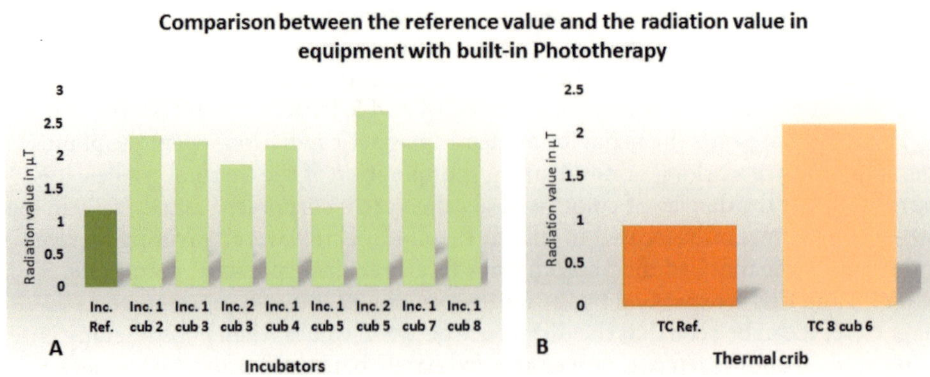

Figure 10.
Comparison graphs of electromagnetic radiation with application of phototherapy in incubator (A) and thermal cradles (B).

accompanied by a level of non-ionizing radiation provided by the electrical components they have the same.

The International Commission for Non-Ionizing Radiation Protection (ICNIRP) maintains a research protocol on non-ionizing radiation that leads to modifying from time to time the recommendations regarding the levels of radiation that can be absorbed by humans, without causing physiological or cellular damage [23].

Electromagnetic fields are waves of energy that exert their effect on the medium they pass through. The ability they have to alter temperature, change polarity, and transform metallic compounds of the periodic table are the tools that are attributed to say that these are capable of causing damage at a physiological and cellular level, especially in the stage where the child is most vulnerable trying to adapt to the postnatal transition. These damages are based on scientific research [24], stating hypotheses such as:

- Appearance of childhood leukemia in the first decade of life, this statement is based on research carried out, in vitro and in vivo. Leukemia is a disease characterized by arrest in the maturation of the cells responsible for the formation of blood constituents, with proliferation and uncontrolled growth of immature blood cells. This proliferation originates at the level of the bone marrow, from which it spreads to the blood and different tissues. If a child receives electromagnetic radiation during the first days of life where the organs are trying to balance the differences between the prenatal and postnatal environment, completion of that maturation may not occur or may occur very slowly. This is because EMFs act on cell membranes by distorting signals from the outside, which are directed to the organelles inside the cell, including the nucleus [25]. This could modify the electrochemical balance of the cells, affecting protein synthesis and causing a distortion of the bioelectric functions of the organism and changes in genetic transmission; which suggests their possible relationship with the development of different types of cancer [26] and alterations in the cellular ionic level caused by the influence of the polarization they induce on the cell membrane.

- Chronic immunology problems and the appearance of different types of cancer before adulthood. Neonates are the most vulnerable people to receive these damages because they are in a stage of development where they do not have the defenses that the mother's womb could provide. It is known that melatonin is the hormone par excellence that regulates sleep cycles and the immune system. It is also an efficient fighter against free radicals that generate cancer cells [27, 28]. This is produced during the part of the day when darkness reigns, and the sun's electromagnetic radiation is attenuated due to the distance between it and the position in which the person is located. In a neonate, there is almost no generation of this hormone in the first weeks of birth, and the body is dedicated to spending the reserves generated by the mother during pregnancy [29, 30]. As long as the child receives electromagnetic radiation through any means in the circadian sleep cycle, melatonin generation does not occur or is deficient, so it cannot fulfill the functions for which it is intended and can cause long-term damage in this regard.

5.4 Recommendations about the use of light in a NICU

The recommendations proposed are aimed at both the use of light for treatment and the use of light in the environmental environment:

- The effectiveness of phototherapy depends on the absorption of light photons by bilirubin molecules [31]. Bilirubin has a yellow pigment, so blue light is the most recommended because bilirubin molecules absorb light photons of this wavelength better than any other. It is recommended to only use blue light, in case of high bilirubin levels, spaced during the day and not at night.

- Although white light has 35% blue and green light in its composition [8], it does not achieve the effectiveness of blue light, so treatment with this type of light, although it may have an effect, would over a long period of time (taking into account that it is only recommended during the day) and the child would be exposed for a prolonged period to the effect of electromagnetic radiation that could cause long-term damage to his or her health.

- The recommended distance for placing the lamps on the RN is 20 to 30 cm. It is requested that review this existing recommendation in the phototherapy protocol because light lamps are magnetic field emitters whose installation standard proposes a minimum distance of 1.5 m from people.

- It is recommended to place lamps in each position occupied by an incubator or thermal crib, so that, if it is necessary to turn them on at night, they do not affect the sleep of other babies.

- If fluorescent lamps are used for general lighting, they must be replaced from time to time to avoid a decrease in visibility when required.

- For general lighting, the use of LED lamps is recommended due to their long life in terms of hours (30,000) and the advantage of not producing heat, which gives them the superiority of increasing irradiance.

6. Conclusions

The use of light in a neonatal intensive care unit is of vital importance for the care of preterm neonates.

Taking into account the characteristics of the composition of visible light is a premise for the efficient use of phototherapy in newborns with conditions at birth.

Keep in mind that artificial light, although it is a tool whose operation depends on electrical energy, is vital for the subsequent state of health of children born with conditions; it provides invisible risks that affect their subsequent development.

Conflict of interest

The authors declare no conflict of interest.

DOI: http://dx.doi.org/10.5772/intechopen.1004454

Author details

Janet Carvajal de la Osa[1*], Yenisel Díaz Roller[1] and Iosvany Aguiar Ramos[2]

1 Universidad Tecnológica de la Habana "José Antonio Echeverría", La Habana, Cuba

2 Centro de Biomateriales de la Universidad de La Habana, La Habana, Cuba

*Address all correspondence to: janetco@automatica.cujae.edu.cu; janetco@gmail.com

References

[1] Rodríguez RG, Pattini AE. Iluminación en unidades de cuidados intensivos neonatales: actualización y recomendaciones. Archivos Argentinos de Pediatría. 2016;**114**(4):361-367. DOI: 10.5546/aap.2016.361

[2] Soto Conti CP. Bilirrubina: mecanismos tóxicos de una molécula antioxidante. Archivos Argentinos de Pediatría. 2021;**119**(1):e18-e25. DOI: 10.5546/aap.2021.e18

[3] Duran M, García JA, Sánchez A. Efectividad de la fototerapia en la hiperbilirrubinemia neonatal. Enfermería Universitaria. 2015;**12**(1): 41-45. DOI: 10.1016/j.reu.2015.05.006

[4] Gabàs MJ. Maxwell: la teoría electromagnética de la luz. Arbor. 2015;**191**(775):a265. DOI: 10.3989/arbor.2015.775n500

[5] Henao Robledo F. In: ECOE Ediciones, editor. Riesgos Físicos II: Iluminación. In: Colección Ingeniería y salud en el trabajo. 2nd ed. 2014. p. 234 consultado en Abril de 2023. Available from: https://books.google.co.ve/books?id=8MK4DQAAQBAJ&printsec=frontcover&hl=es#v=onepage&q&f=false

[6] del Mazo VA, Velasco Maillo S, García-Molina R. Recomposición de un rayo de luz blanca descompuesto por un prisma. Eureka sobre Enseñanza y Divulgación de las Ciencias. 2020;**17**(3):340201-340209 https://doi.org/10.25267/Rev_Eureka_ensen_divulg_cienc.2020.v17.i3.3402

[7] Mosquera Torres AM, Basto Guevara JA, Reyes Domínguez JF. La popular luz azul: ¿por qué es nociva para la salud visual? Ámbito Investigativo. 2020;**5**(2):72-80. Available from: https://ciencia.lasalle.edu.co/ai

[8] Boulton ME, Brainard GC, Jones W, Karpecki P, Melton R, Thomas R. Blue light hazard: New knowledge, new approaches to maintaining ocular health. In: Points de Vue - International Review of Ophthalmic Optics; Report of a roundtable 16 march 2013. New York city, USA: Essilor International; 2015. pp. 2-12. Available from: www.ko-go.org.tr

[9] Jiménez-Rubio G, Solís-Chagoyán H, Domínguez-Alonso A, Benítez-King G. Alteraciones del ciclo circadiano en las enfermedades psiquiátricas: papel sincronizador de la melatonina en el ciclo sueño-vigilia y la polaridad neuronal. Salud Mental. 2011;**34**:167-173. Available from:https://www.scielo.org.mx/scielo.php?script=sci_arttext&pid=S0185-33252011000200010

[10] Jeffrey MM, AF MD. Fototerapia para la ictericia neonatal. Revista del Hospital Materno Infantil Ramón Sardá. 2008;**27**(3):100-111. Available from:https://www.redalyc.org/articulo.oa?id=91227302

[11] Sadowska M, Narbutt J, Lesiak A. Blue light in dermatology. Life. 2021;**11**(7):670. DOI: 10.3390/life11070670

[12] Ruiz Sánchez JG, de León FB, González Pérez-de Villar N, Gomes Porras M, Herranz de la Morena L. Niveles de bilirrubina como predictor favorable en la diabetes mellitus Tipo 2. In: XXIX Congreso Nacional De La Sociedad Española De Diabetes, Oviedo, 18-20 de abril de 2018. Endocrinología, Diabetes y Nutrición. 2018;**65**(Espec Cong 1):79. Available from: https://static.elsevier.es›congresos ›pdf›cong_sed2018

[13] Slaughter JL, Kemper AR, Newman TB. Technical report: Diagnosis and management of hyperbilirubinemia

in the newborn infant 35 or more weeks of gestation. Pediatrics. 2022;**150**(3):e2022058865. DOI: 10.1542/peds.2022-058865

[14] Faulhaber FRS, Procianoy RS, Silveira RC. Side effects of phototherapy on neonates. American Journal of Perinatology. 2019;**36**(3):252-257. DOI: 10.1055/s-0038-1667379

[15] Newman TB, Wu YW, Kuzniewicz MW, et al. Childhood seizures after phototherapy. Pediatrics. 2018;**142**(4):e20180648. DOI: 10.1542/peds.2018-0648

[16] Boidi, del artículo C. Efectos secundarios de la luminoterapia en neonatos. Revista Enfermería Neonatal. 2019;**31**:38-42. Available from:https://riu.austral.edu.ar/handle/123456789/1016

[17] García del Río M, Sánchez Luna M, Doménech Martínez E, et al. Revisión de los estándares y recomendaciones para el diseño de una unidad de neonatología. Anales de Pediatría (Barcelona, Spain). 2007;**67**(6):594-602. DOI: 10.1016/S1695-4033(07)70810-X

[18] de la Rosa Castillo MJ. Análisis de los cambios de coloración cuantificados por colorimetría en la piel de recién nacidos expuestos a fototerapía. Tesis para obtener el diploma de la Especialidad en Pediatría. San Luis Potosí: Universidad Autónoma de San Luis Potosí; 2020

[19] Pickler R, McGrath J, Reyna B, Tubbs-Cooley H, Best AI, et al. Effects of the neonatal intensive care unit environment on preterm infant oral feeding. Research and Reports in Neonatology. 2013;**2013**(3):15-20. DOI: 10.2147/RRN.S41280

[20] Riad SM, Salama IM. Electromagnetic Fields and Waves Fundamentals of Engineering. McGraw-Hill Education; 2020. p. 688 consultado en mayo de 2023. Available from: https://www.mhprofessional.com/electromagnetic-fields-and-waves-fundamentals-of-engineering-9781260457148-usa

[21] Council of the European Union. Council Recommendation of 12 July 1999 on the Limitation of Exposure of the General Public to Electromagnetic Fields (0 Hz to 300 GHz). Brussels, Belgium: Official Journal of the European Communities; July 1999

[22] International Agency for Research on Cancer (IARC). Non-ionizing Radiation, Part 1: Static and Extremely Low-frequency (ELF) Electric and Magnetic Fields. In: IARC Monographs on the Evaluation of Carcinogenic Risks to Humans. Vol. 80. Lyon, France; 2002. p. 445 ISBN 92 832 1280 0

[23] ICNIRP. Guidelines for limiting exposure to time-varying electric and magnetic fields (1 Hz - 100 kHz). Health Physics. 2010;**99**(6):818-836. DOI: 10.1097/HP.0b013e3181f06c86

[24] Moon JH. Health effects of electromagnetic fields on children. Clinical and Experimental Pediatrics. 2020;**63**(11):422-428. DOI: 10.3345/cep.2019.01494

[25] Brabant C, Geerinck A, Beaudart C, Tirelli E, Geuzaine C, Bruyere O. Exposure to magnetic fields and childhood leukemia: A systematic review and meta-analysis of casecontrol and cohort studie. Reviews on Environmental Health. 2021;**38**(2):1-12. DOI: 10.1515/reveh-2021-0112

[26] Seomun G, Lee J, Park J. Exposure to extremely low-frequency magnetic fields and childhood cancer: A systematic review and meta-analysis. PLoS One. 2021;**16**(5):e0251628. DOI: 10.1371/journal.pone.0251628

[27] Reiter RJ, Manchester LC, Dun-Xian T. Neurotoxins: Free radical mechanisms and melatonin protection. Current Neuropharmacology. 2010;**8**(3):194-210. DOI: 10.2174/157015910792246236

[28] Hacışevki A y Baba B. An overview of melatonin as an antioxidant molecule: A biochemical approach. In: Melatonin Drăgoi CM, Nicolae AC, editors. Intech Open; 2018. DOI:10.5772/intechopen.79421

[29] Carvajal de la Osa J, Santana GJ, Herrera GM, Sánchez GA, Pérez Almirall I. Campo magnético ambiental en una Unidad de Terapia Intensiva Neonatal. Importancia de su verificación. Archivos Argentinos de Pediatría. 2020;**118**(3):e246-e251. DOI: 10.5546/aap.2020.e246

[30] Muñoz Hoyos A, Bonillo Perales A, Ávila-Villegas R, González-Ripoll M, et al. Melatonin levels during the first week of life and their relation with the antioxidant response in the perinatal period. Neonatology. 2007;**92**(3):209-216. DOI: 10.1159/000102957

[31] Ávila Reyes R, Suárez Llanas BA, Pérez Abrego CE, Masud Yunes-Zárraga JL, et al. Luz emitida por diodo (LED) en el tratamiento de la hiperbilirrubinemia neonatal. Un prototipo de fototerapia a bajo costo hecho en México. Pediatría de México. 2013;**15**(3):73-79. Available from: https://1library.co/document/dzx1e4oy-emitida-diodo-tratamiento-hiperbilirrubinemia-neonatal-prototipo-fototerapia-mxico.html

Chapter 7

Pain Control

Azamolmolouk Elsagh and Alireza Jashni Motlagh

Abstract

Some studies show that each newborn suffers daily from 16 to 35 painful procedures in their hospitalization. Some of these procedures are IV line access, heel stick, intubation, ET tube suctioning, NG lavage, diaper change, repositioning, and minor surgeries such as circumcision. As neonates cannot reflect their pain obviously, we should use attitude and physiologic responses to triggers for pain assessment. These physiologic responses consist of increasing heart rate and blood pressure, intensity of crying, gesture, desaturation, sweating, immune responses, flexion of extremities, change in ICP, increasing catecholamines. Attitude reflections consist of muscle spasms, insomnia, grimaces, change in circadian cycle. The goal of pain relief is to help the newborn adapt to the created circumstance and reduce stress during the procedure. Pain relief can be achieved by pharmaceutical and non-pharmaceutical methods (e.g., surgery) or a combination of these methods based on the specific needs and goals of each patient. Some of the non-pharmaceutical management are sucrose, swaddling, facilitated tucking, Kangaroo Mother Care (KMC), Non Nutritive Sucking, positioning, massage, breastfeeding. Pharmacologic management consists of non-opioid analgesia and opioid analgesia. All of these methods can reduce the pain of newborns and give them a higher quality of life.

Keywords: neonate, pain, non-opioid analgesia, opioid analgesia, Kangaroo mother care (KMC)

1. Introduction

The goal of pain relief is to help the neonate adapt to the circumstance and reduce stress during the procedure, so it is important to know and manage the pain procedures. Studies showed that some problems with the best management of pain are due to the unawareness of medical workers of assessment tools and the best way of pain control.

As the researchers want to show and control of any pain in neonates, this review has been collected by the authors. This chapter consists of two parts, pharmaceutical and non-pharmaceutical (massage and breast milk) pain relief, which have been described in detail for readers.

At the end of this chapter, the reader is expected to:

1. Learn various pain relief methods.

2. Become familiar with non-pharmaceutical pain relief methods in neonates.

3. Know the benefits of non-pharmaceutical pain relief methods.

4. Become encouraged to use non-pharmaceutical pain relief methods in the intensive care unit.

2. Pain management in neonates

Based on the knowledge of recent years, it was thought that neonates have no sense of pain because of myelin deficiency in their nerve fibers and they had many surgeries without any anesthesia, but now a day we know that this defect only causes the retarded transferring of pain signal. Some studies show that each newborn suffers daily from many painful procedures in their hospitalization. As neonates cannot reflect their pain obviously, we should use attitude and physiologic responses to triggers for pain assessment.

Short-term outcomes of pain are change in the circadian cycle, attitude change till 22 hours after a painful procedure, more excitability to following pain, intraventricular hemorrhage, persistent crying, difficulty in falling in asleep, delayed wound healing, changes in immunity, bonding defect, biochemical changes such as hyperglycemia, increasing protein catabolism, increase in cortisol, catecholamine, glucagon, growth hormone, renin, aldosterone, ADH and decrease of insulin.

Long-term outcomes include neurodevelopmental delay, different responses to the same triggers, long-term changes in neurotransmitters, and brain damage. So it is important to know and manage the pain procedures. Studies showed that some problems with the best management of pain are due to the unawareness of medical workers of assessment tools and the best way of pain control.

This chapter will provide these orientations to us.

3. Results and discussion

Pain relief planning for neonates can be accomplished by a multidisciplinary team consisting of doctors, nurses, physiotherapists, and, most importantly, the family. Attention should be paid to the specific role of each member of this team in relieving the newborn's pain and causing him/her to relax, as well as cooperation and collaboration between the team members and showing enthusiasm in relieving the baby's pain. Each member of the team may have his/her own unique strategy for detecting and alleviating the baby's pain, making the coordination between these members and the application of every single method a challenge, which must be discussed before starting the treatment in order to prepare a precise therapeutic plan. Therefore, it is more appropriate to review applicable pain relief methods before starting the treatment and preparing therapeutic plans.

The goal of pain relief is to help the newborn adapt to the created circumstance and reduce stress during the procedure. Pain relief can be achieved by pharmaceutical and non-pharmaceutical methods (e.g., surgery) or a combination of these methods based on the specific needs and goals of each patient. Each of these methods can affect different neuronal pathways involved in pain perception [1].

4. Pharmaceutical pain reduction methods in neonates

The type of pharmaceutical treatment varies depending on the source and severity of the pain, as well as the level of discomfort and side effects of the method.

4.1 Non-opioid analgesia

Aspirin, acetaminophen, ibuprofen, and naproxen can relieve mild to moderate local pain. For neonates that cannot tolerate oral drugs, Ketorolac can be administered intravenously. The dosage is 20–25 mg/kg of body weight for oral acetaminophen and 30 mg/kg when the drug is delivered via the rectal pathway.

4.2 Opioid analgesia

This category of drugs suppresses pain without affecting consciousness and includes opioid analgesics that act on synaptic transporters in different parts of the central nervous system by binding to natural narcotics in the body. These drugs may either block the ascending pain signals in the posterior horn of the spinal cord by affecting the basal ganglia and activating the descending path of pain or cause the pain to become bearable by creating a sensory response to pain through the limbic system.

These drugs include morphine, methadone, pentazocine, propoxyphene, fentanyl, fentanyl citrate, oxycodone, and codeine. The effect of morphine starts only 5 minutes after administration and lasts for up to 15 minutes; however, if this agent is used without a painful stimulus, it may imperil the life of cells (**Table 1**) [2].

Name of drugs	Indication	Dosage and routes of administration	Complications	Consideration
Fentanyl	Sedation/ analgesia, Anesthesia	0.5–4 mcg/kg Sedation/ analgesia per dose IV slow push Infusion rate: 1–5 mcg/kg/h. 5–50 mcg/kg: Anesthesia	Respiratory depression, Chest wall rigidity, Urinary problems	Naloxone should be available
Methadone	Opiate withdrawal management	Primary dose: 0.05–0.2 mg/kg every 12–24 h then wean dose 10–20% each week till 4–6 weeks	Respiratory depression, Ileus, Delayed gastric emptying, Long QT interval	Cardiac monitoring, accurate dose decreasing
Morphine	Sedation/ analgesia, Opiate withdrawal management	0.05–0.02 mg/kg IV over at least 5 min Start with continuous infusion of 100–150 mcg/kg Till 1 h and then 10–20 mcg/kg/h. Oral dose: 0.03–0.1 mg/kg per dose orally every 3–4 h; wean dose 10–20% every 2/3 days	Respiratory depression, Ileus, Abdominal distention, Urinary problems	Naloxone should be available

Table 1.
Narcotic usage in neonates.

4.3 Local anesthetics

This group of painkillers acts on the cell membrane and disrupts the elevation of the permeability of sodium channels on the axon membrane, a phenomenon that usually occurs after depolarization, preventing the dissemination of the action potential along the axon. Examples of these agents include lidocaine, prilocaine, bupivacaine, chloroprocaine, and tetracaine. Lidocaine and bupivacaine solutions (1– 0.5%) are used in infants at a continuous intravenous infusion dose of 0.2 mg/kg/h. If there is a need for local anesthesia, a dose of 0.5 mL/kg is applicable.

Emla cream contains 2.5% lidocaine and 2.3% prilocaine, and 1–2 g of this cream can be applied for 60–90 minutes prior to vein puncture and painful procedures such as circumcision. Each gram of Emla cream contains 25 mg of lidocaine and 25 mg of prilocaine.

4.4 Regional anesthetics

Anesthetics can sometimes be used as regional blockers, which are applied for nerve blocks via epidural/caudal, dorsal, or intercostal routes. This strategy can be useful in reducing the systemic effects of drugs, particularly when narcotics have led to respiratory complications and apnea. Spinal block is applicable in surgeries below the navel, and epidural/caudal block is used during thoracic, abdominal, and limb surgeries. This type of anesthesia is associated with the risk of incomplete block or neuronal damage, and therefore, it should be performed by appropriately trained anesthesiologists. Today, ultrasound-guided insertion of a needle containing the anesthetic agent offers a novel technique that demands special skills and needs more investigations before it can be recommended for infants.

5. Non-pharmaceutical methods

Studies show the effectiveness of simple non-pharmaceutical methods in relieving pain symptoms. Recently, there has been great emphasis on non-pharmaceutical and non-surgical methods of pain relief as preferable strategies. In premature neonates, non-pharmaceutical methods such as reducing light and noise in the environment and behavioral supports can help mitigate restlessness and reduce the need for painkillers. Furthermore, care training for healthcare staff and parents, including repositioning, sleep regulation, playing music, soft touching, shaking, and non-nutritional sucking, can be effective in reducing stress and the response to pain. Other methods in this area include music therapy, touch therapy, massage, thermal therapy, cryotherapy, aromatherapy, feeding with sucrose and breast milk, etc. In the following, a number of non-pharmaceutical methods frequently suggested for pain control in neonates have been described [3].

5.1 Sucrose

Sucrose is a sweet disaccharide (glucose + fructose) that, by affecting taste receptors located on the tip of the tongue, can trigger the release of intrinsic opioids; however, this agent is not effective when it is administered by injection. Feeding with 2 mL of oral sucrose solution 2 minutes prior to painful procedures has been very helpful in reducing procedural pains. Various studies have shown that oral sucrose has been much more effective than Emla cream, even in premature neonates. Due to the high cost of this agent in our country, it has been recommended that 10% glucose can be a viable alternative with the same efficacy [4].

5.2 Facilitated tucking

In this method, a sheet or a thin blanket is thrown over the baby lying on the bed or inside the nest so that the baby's organs are completely covered. This method is different from swaddling because it does not restrict the baby's limb movements.

5.3 Swaddling

This is a very beneficial way to pacify the newborn, especially those older than 31 weeks. In this method, the neonate is completely wrapped in a thin quadrilateral blanket so that only one hand is out of the swaddle. This method is particularly effective in babies who suffer from maternal deprivation syndrome. Also, cuddling babies is facilitated by this method (**Figure 1**).

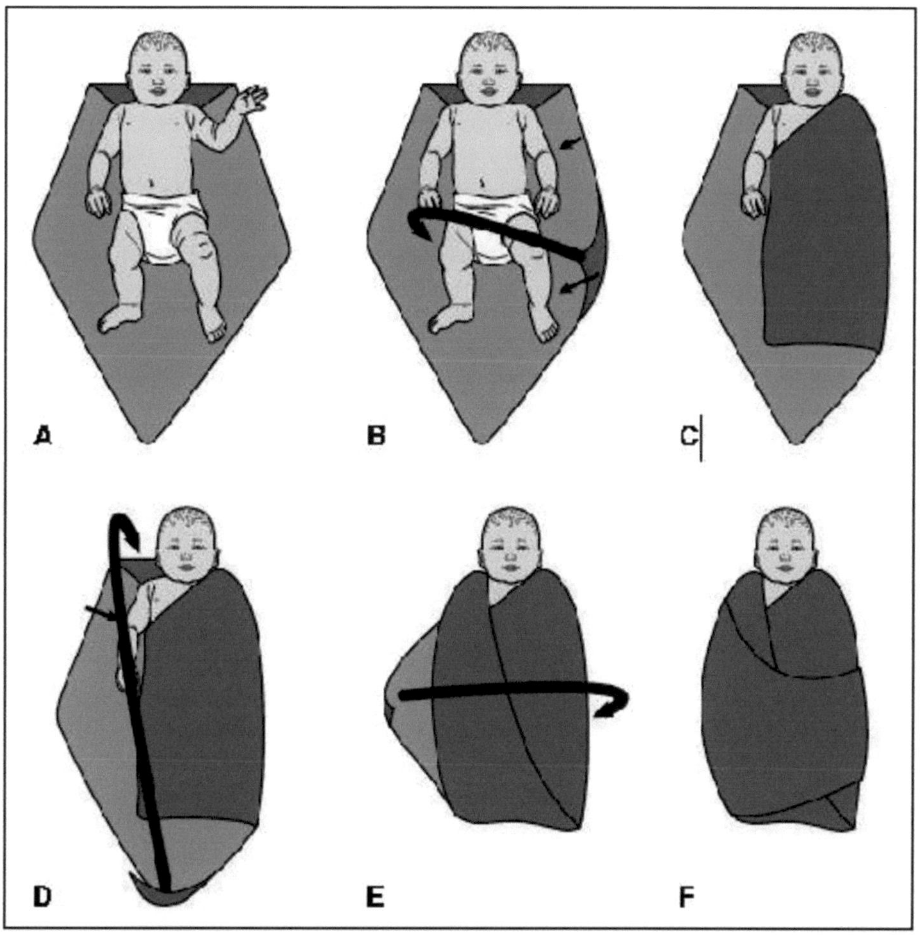

Figure 1.
Method of swaddling. Adopted with permission from clinical handbook of neonatal pain management for nurses, 1st edition, Tara Marko, Michele Dickson, 2016.

5.4 Kangaroo mother care

In 1978 at the Materno Society in Santa, Rey and Martinez presented kangaroo mother care (KMC) as a method recommended for caring for infants. The term KMC is derived from the kangaroo mother care method, where the mother acts as an incubator, and the main nutritional source for the preterm low-birth-weight (LBW) neonates, and the extrauterine life conditions allow the baby to grow similar to term neonates. In KMC, the baby only wears diapers, allowing for direct skin-to-skin contact with the mother, and then a thin bedsheet is laid on them. During KMC, it is better for the mother to sit on a sofa at a 60° angle. This method provides prolonged and continuous touching between the mother and the newborn in the hospital and after discharge and can boost the neonate's desire for feeding. The KMC method regulates the heart and respiratory rates, deepens sleep, reduces crying and risk of nosocomial infections, improves weight gain and height growth, increases feeding with breast milk, reduces postpartum depression, and also boosts parental satisfaction with the treatment process.

This is also a very effective method in reducing procedural pain in the hospital. In this area, various studies have affirmed the effectiveness of this method in alleviating pain during blood sampling from the heel. In addition, this method can be used in neonates connected to a ventilator or Nasal Continues Positive Airway Pressure (NCPAP).

5.4.1 Objectives of KMC

- Boosting newborns' physical health, especially in premature babies;
- Improving the growth and development of the infants hospitalized in the neonatal intensive care unit;
- Lowering the levels of stress, depression, and feeling guilty and increasing parents' self-confidence and abilities while taking care of their premature babies;
- Improving the methods of care provision to premature newborns in the hospital and at home;
- Nurturing the emotional attachment between the newborn and the parents;
- Reducing the duration of hospitalization of the neonate;
- Optimizing the use of manpower and technology in the neonatal intensive care unit;
- Reducing the rates of nosocomial infections and mortality in hospitals;
- Empowering the parents of premature babies to deeply engage them as their babies' caretakers;
- Encouraging feeding with breast milk for premature babies and familiarizing parents with different methods of breastfeeding;
- Creating a care team with the participation of parents in order to deliver more effective family-oriented care.

5.4.2 Benefits of KMC

Breastfeeding: The KMC method, not only during hospitalization but also after discharge, can encourage exclusive breastfeeding and increase breast milk production.

Control of body temperature and metabolism: Studies show that KMC, in comparison with incubator care, can better maintain the normal body temperature in neonates, preventing hypothermia and causing faster warming of hypothermic neonates.

Resolving newborns' problems: It has been noted that the KMC method reduces vomiting, respiratory problems, infections, crying, etc., in neonates.

Positive effects on the five senses: The KMC method strengthens the neonate's five main senses. The newborn senses the warmth of the mother's body through skin-to-skin contact (touch), listens to the mother's voice and heartbeat (auditory), sucks the mother's breasts (taste), makes eye contact with the mother (vision), and perceives the mother's smells (olfactory).

Growth improvement: The KMC method causes the baby to gain weight better.

Psychological effects: The KMC care technique is beneficial not only to the neonate but also to the parents. By KMC, mothers feel less stressed compared to when the baby is developing in an incubator. Also, mothers seem to prefer skin-to-skin contact to conventional care, believing that this approach augments their relaxation, self-confidence, feeling capable, and self-satisfaction as they feel satisfied with the fact that they can do something for their premature babies. Generally, fathers also feel more relaxed, comfortable, and attached during KMC care. In addition, these newborns are more likely to possess positive social personalities in the future.

Health staff's reduction of workload: The advantages of KMC is that it obviates the need for hiring additional employees by establishing a family-oriented care unit overwhelmed with scientific and emotional relationships.

Reduction of neonatal mortality rate: Numerous studies have shown that KMC is associated with a reduction in the mortality of premature babies.

5.4.3 Implementing KMC

5.4.3.1 Skin-to-skin contact

This part includes the direct and long-term (1 hour at first and for longer periods thereafter) contact of the mother's skin with the baby's skin, which should be accomplished as soon as possible after birth [5].

5.4.3.2 Physical, emotional, and educational support

The mother, father, and family should be supported by doctors, nurses, midwives, and medical staff. Moreover, receiving support from the community, family, and spouse is particularly needed.

5.4.3.3 Exclusive breastfeeding

This step encompasses supporting and encouraging exclusive feeding with breastmilk, either directly from the mother's breast or using extracted breastmilk via auxiliary tools such as gastric tubes, syringes, cups, spoons, etc. Most babies weighing below 1500 grams start to gain weight desirably after being exclusively fed with breastmilk.

5.4.3.4 Early discharge and then follow-ups

When KMC care starts in the hospital, it will lead to the early discharge of the premature baby. This type of care can then continue at home. After discharge and in order to ensure the health condition of the baby, parents should refer to the hospital based on a pre-scheduled follow-up plan.

5.4.4 Who can benefit from KMC?

All newborns can receive KMC; however, extremely premature babies requiring special care need to be placed inside a radiant warmer and an incubator, and KMC can be postponed until the neonate's condition is stabilized.

Birth weight of 1800 g or higher: If the condition of the neonate is stabilized, KMC can be delivered immediately after birth.

Birth weight of 1200–1800 g: In such cases, labor should be performed in well-equipped facilities possessing requirements for newborn care. Otherwise, the baby and the mother should be transferred to the NICU immediately after birth so that advanced care and KMC can be initiated. One of the best ways to transfer the newborn is to carry him/her while having skin-to-skin contact with the mother.

Birth weight equal to or lower than 1200 g: These babies should be transferred to a well-equipped hospital with advanced newborn care facilities before birth. In these cases, days or weeks may be required before the baby's condition allows for delivering KMC. Mortality and complications are substantially high in these babies, and they should be transferred to a level 3 healthcare center to receive special care.

5.4.5 Noteworthy issues about KMC

Being eligible for receiving KMC depends on several factors. In most cases, birth weight alone can predict who can benefit from this type of care.

Overall, a birth weight of >1200 g is considered suitable for receiving KMC if the following items are met:

1. An intrauterine age of at least 30 weeks based on LMP and 28 weeks based on the time of fertilization.

2. The baby's having a stable hemodynamic condition under mechanical ventilation (if applicable).

3. The baby's being kept inside an incubator or a cut.

4. Babies under the radiant heating device may not be ready for KMC. The use of a warmer device shows that she/he is not yet in a completely stable condition, requiring additional interventions to stabilize the clinical condition.

5.4.6 Step-by-step performing of KMC

- Before starting, the mother should consider personal preparations such as emptying the bladder.

- The mother's body temperature should be measured.

- Appropriate ambient temperature should be between 21 and 24°C.
- The baby's armpit temperature should be measured, and if it is within the normal and acceptable range, KMC can be initiated.
- Necessary tools should be prepared.
- A warm and soft four-layer bedsheet should be provided so that if it becomes hot, the thickness can be reduced by removing layers.
- A comfortable chair should be provided.
- A pulse oximeter should be provided (optional).
- Underfoot should be provided.
- Small pillows, as needed, should be provided for the mother's comfort.
- Thermometer for check the temperature.
- Appropriate clothing for KMC regarding the local culture, the mother's comfort, and the baby's safety.
- Hat (mandatory for babies weighing less than 1500 g), socks, diapers, and open-front clothes (when the ambient temperature falls below 22°C).
- A mirror to see the baby (optional).

5.4.7 Contraindications of KMC

- Neonates who are clinically unstable and have fluctuating arterial blood oxygen saturation.
- Neonates who have an arterial catheter or chest tube.
- Neonates who are predisposed to intraventricular bleeding.
- Neonates who receive vasopressor and inotrope drugs.
- Neonates bearing a central venous catheter in the shoulder area.
- Neonates who suffer from respiratory instability or are under mechanical ventilation.
- Babies who have become suddenly ill within 24 hours.
- Babies who suffer from persistent apnea and bradycardia require respiratory stimulation.
- Parents suffering from cutaneous lesions or ulcers or acute illnesses should postpone this type of care until complete recovery.

- Parents who have abnormal physical and mental conditions.
- Parents who have not received the necessary training and skills in this field.

5.4.8 The following items should be paid attention to when delivering KMC at home

- The ambient temperature should be kept at 21–22°C for term babies and 22–24°C for premature babies.
- Although it is easy to perform KMC at home, it requires sufficient skill and knowledge.
- The mother can perform her daily work at the same time.
- At home, the mother should be encouraged to perform exercise and mental relaxation to achieve peace.
- The mother must be familiar with the different methods of breastfeeding a premature baby and acquire the necessary skills at the hospital.
- The mother can provide KMC care in a half-seated or half-lying position (on a bed or a chair).

5.5 Cradle rocking

Gently rocking the baby can be very effective in reducing procedural pain. It seems that the mother's comfortably sitting on a rolling chair while providing KMC can also be very helpful. A study by Amon *et al.* in 2014 showed that pain scores and maternal stress were significantly reduced when mothers cuddled their infants and whispered to them.

5.6 Non-nutritive sucking

Non-nutritive sucking refers to placing a pacifier in the baby's mouth (i.e., sucking without feeding). According to the valve control theory, the mechanical effect of sucking includes prevention from the transmission of pain impulses to the brain. According to this theory, if either pain is not recognized by the brain or pain signal transmission to the brain is blocked, the negative consequences of pain will disappear. Recent studies conducted on the effect of non-nutritive sucking with sucrose on pain have indicated that the combined use of these methods considerably reduces pain.

5.7 Position

Holding the baby, especially the preterm infant, in its natural position can help reduce pain. Infants tend to be in their fetal position, so they can be supported in such positions with the help of swaddling and tools such as a strap.

5.8 Surroundings

Management of the environment can include reducing the light and noise, avoiding the manipulation of the baby, and managing the sleep-wake cycle, all of which aim to increase relaxation and reduce pain.

5.9 Massage

Throughout history, humans have been using massage to alleviate pain and enhance healing. Massage was first practiced more than 5000 years ago in China and Mesopotamia and is one of the oldest health practices. In 1894, the Association of Trained Massage Therapists was formed, and modern massage therapy techniques were developed worldwide and used for rehabilitation by 1900.

Massage means hitting with the hand and rubbing an organ when a person feels pain or injury. These are almost automatic movements. Cops *et al*. quoted Freeman (2004), noting that massage could improve health and heal the body and mind. Massage therapy is an integrated part of health in hospitals, nursing homes, and other health centers. Massage therapy is a curative technique in which the therapist, through focused awareness, uses his hands as a focal point to create balance and harmony regarding the bilateral patient-environment energy field.

Over the years, studies on massage therapy have revealed the pain-reducing effects of this technique, accompanied by increased blood and lymph flow within superficial lymphatic capillaries and improved respiratory function due to the removal of mucus from the respiratory tract.

Massage primarily facilitates blood flow. When muscles are rubbed and subjected to tension, they expedite blood return to the heart, driving acids such as lactic acid out of the muscle tissue. In addition, improved blood flow enhances tissue perfusion and oxygenation. Massage also induces the release of endorphins (i.e., natural analgesics) in the body.

5.9.1 Evidence on the effects of massage therapy

Recently, a systematic review on the role of tactile stimulation in healthy infants revealed that massage during infancy might have beneficial effects on sleep and crying patterns, neonatal stress levels, circadian rhythms, mother-infant interaction, and neonatal development and well-being.

5.9.2 Massage and procedural pain

Infants are likely to experience one of the numerous painful procedures while receiving routine health care, such as heel blood sampling heel, circumcisions, and vaccination. These painful procedures during infancy and childhood may influence the child's response to pain in the future. In studies on the infants undergoing heel blood sampling, fewer facial expressions and a lower increase in the heart rate were observed in the infants receiving massage compared to their peers in the control group [6].

5.9.3 Massage in low-birth-weight infants

Various studies (n = 14) have reported that massage can reduce hospital stays and improve weight gain. In LBW neonates, massage can improve sleep quality, reduce stress behaviors, enhance vagal activity and gastrointestinal tract movements, and increase the levels of insulin and insulin-like growth factors.

There is ample evidence supporting the beneficial effects of massage therapy on anxiety, depression, complications of autism spectrum disorders, chemotherapy side effects, diabetes symptoms, rheumatoid arthritis pain, and pulmonary function in adults and, to a lesser extent, in children; however, there are no such studies on neonates.

Five basic techniques are used in massage therapy, including:

1. Floorage

2. Petrissage

3. Friction

4. Tapotement

5. Vibration

Ling and Mezger defined floorage as stroking, which is a movement during which the hand slides over the skin without moving the deep muscles. Also, petrissage is a rubbing and pressing movement where the muscles are grasped and raised by the hand. This movement mitigates muscle pain by discarding lactic acid and boosting muscular blood flow. During friction, the masseur uses the thumbs and other fingertips to work around the joints, as well as the thickest parts of the muscles.

In the tapotement technique, the masseur uses the margins of the hands, fingers, and palms (formed as cup-like) to introduce tiny, professional, and strip movements. Generally, tapotement refers to any rapid and consecutive tapping aiming to stimulate the local blood flow and induce hyperemia, as well as prolonged tapping leading to muscle exhaustion and relaxation.

During vibration, the therapist's open hands are firmly placed on the muscle, leading to rapid local vibrations for several seconds. This movement continues until the entire muscle vibrates and helps stimulate the nervous system, boosting blood flow and improving endocrine function.

5.9.4 Mechanism of action of massage therapy

The mechanism of action of massage therapy has not been fully understood in children, infants, or adults. One hypothesis suggests that massage therapy may promote biochemical changes in soft tissues, including elevated blood flow and oxygenation of muscles and connective tissues. Recent studies have proposed that massage can increase the level of oxytocin hormone and nurture a feeling of well-being, leading to a reduction in anxiety. The pain-relieving effects of massage therapy may also be due to the secretion of endorphins and serotonin. Another hypothesis states that massage can stimulate thick neuronal fibers, suppressing the thin neuronal fibers interacting with pain receptors, which exactly mimics the valve control mechanism [7].

5.9.5 Benefits of massage therapy

1. Alleviating procedural pains;

2. Reducing anxiety and depression;

3. Reducing stress;

4. Improving weight gain in premature neonates;
5. Reducing the risk of autism in premature neonates;
6. Improving pulmonary function;
7. Relaxation and stabilization of vital signs;
8. Reducing cardiac dysrhythmias;
9. Accelerating the healing of bone fractures;
10. Improving tension headaches;
11. Treatment of anemia;
12. Acceleration of wound healing;
13. Reducing joint pain and improving joint function in neonates suffering from degenerative arthritis and osteoarthritis.

5.10 Breastfeeding and breast milk

Aside from the methods already mentioned, breastfeeding is one of the physiological methods of pain reduction in infants. The benefits of breastfeeding are numerous. Breastfeeding has significantly reduced morbidity and mortality during infancy and childhood worldwide and has contributed to the health of communities beyond perceptions and expectations. Studies have shown that infants breastfed enjoy numerous short-term and long-term benefits due to the presence of a variety of essential biomolecules in breast milk. On the other hand, infants who remain deprived of milk or breast milk generally require costly treatments in the hospital.

The infant benefits not only from the breast milk itself but also from the mechanical action of breastfeeding. The infant should completely open his/her mouth and place the tongue in the lower part of the lower gum in order to breastfeed effectively. While the tongue remains in this position, a wave-like movement starts along the length of the tongue (from the tip to the bottom). The breast tissue is placed inside the infant's mouth, and due to the pressure caused by the wave-like movement against the breast tissues facing the hard palate, milk starts to pour out from its reserves (lactiferous sinuses) into the infant's throat, where the act of swallowing takes place. So, it seems that the sucking actions taking place to squeeze out milk from the mother's breasts can optimally exercise the soft palate muscles.

Some of these factors inevitably interfere with effective oral feeding; nevertheless, breastfeeding is easier to establish and succeed than bottle feeding. Coordination between reflexes, sucking, swallowing, and breathing may be influenced by severe prematurity or underlying diseases.

Multiple studies have declared that breastfeeding affects the response to pain in a sensory-oral way. Also, it has been reported that breastfeeding is one of the natural ways to reduce pain depending on skin-to-skin contact, sucking, and the sweetness of the milk. Recent studies have noted that special and pleasant flavors can reduce pain in neonates. Breast milk (less than 2 mL), along with its proteins, fats, and sweeteners, can effectively lower pain and spontaneous crying in human and mouse infants.

5.10.1 The role of nurses in reducing pain in neonates

It is critical for nurses to intervene in treating pain and preventing its short- and long-term complications in neonates exposed to severe and recurring pain. Regarding professional ethics, nurses are responsible for recognizing and alleviating pain in newborns who are inevitably exposed to pain or in those who are under intubation and unable to express pain by crying. Compared to others, nurses are closer to hospitalized patients, placing them in the best position for detecting, preventing, and treating pain.

5.10.2 Action mechanisms of non-pharmaceutical analgesics

Several mechanisms are presumed for the analgesic effects of non-pharmaceutical pain-relieving interventions. One hypothesis that probably is true for all of these methods considers the valve control theory proposed by Malzak and Wall, according to which stimuli that pass through the ascending routes can suppress pain signal receptors following painful stimuli by employing various intrinsic pathways related to the thalamus of the spinal cord. The stronger these competitive stimuli are, including in the case of multifaceted methods, the more effective they can be in pain perception inhibition. This theory explains why multifaceted interventions, such as kangaroo care, breastfeeding, or sensory saturation (involving tactile, auditory, and olfactory mechanisms) are more effective than individual stimuli (e.g., auditory or olfactory alone). Another mechanism for pain reduction engages the upper parts of the brain and is related to the release of endorphins. Endorphins are released following stress (including pain) or positive stimuli such as touching. For instance, sucrose, due to its sweetness, is believed to induce the release of endorphins. On the other hand, sucking seems to involve mechanical routes (according to valve control theory) in order to prevent the transmission of pain impulses to the brain. According to this theory, the negative consequence of pain wanes if the pain is not perceived by the brain or the transmission of pain signals to the brain is blocked. For various painful procedures, the respective pain-relieving measures can be categorized as noted so that the newborn can benefit from an appropriate palliative treatment (**Table 2**).

5.10.3 Necessary recommendations for better pain management in neonatal intensive care units

- A written clinical guide should be present in every neonatal intensive care unit (NICU), and specific palliative measures should be presented for every painful procedure.
- Non-pharmaceutical pain-reducing methods, such as kangaroo care, swaddling, nesting, oral sucrose, and massage, should be performed in NICUs.
- One should try to eliminate stressful stimuli (auditory, vision, touch, and balance), especially light and excessive noise, in NICUs.
- If applicable, blood sampling should be from the heel.
- In order to reduce pain during catheterization, the specific clinical guide of the same catheter should be used.
- All healthcare workers are required to pass courses on neonatal pain reduction and be aware of the dire consequences of failing to relieve procedural pain.

Management	Analgesia-anesthesia	Opiate analgesia	Oral sucrose	Emla cream	Non-pharmacologic pain relief
Heal stick			×		×
Venipuncture			×	×	×
Intramuscular or Subcutaneous injection			×		×
IV cannulation		×	×	×	×
Arterial puncture & peripheral arterial line			×	×	×
Umbilical catheterization			×		×
Lumbar puncture, Arterial or Venus cut down			×	×	×
Peripherally inserted central catheter	×	×	×	×	×

Table 2.
Classification of pain control in any painful procedure in neonatal ward.

6. Conclusion

At the end of this chapter, authors hope that they can present a qualified program to pain management of newborns and give them a higher quality of life.

Author details

Azamolmolouk Elsagh* and Alireza Jashni Motlagh
Department of Neonatology, Alborz University of Medical Sciences, Karaj, Iran

*Address all correspondence to: a_elsagh@abzums.ac.ir

References

[1] Shepherd TB, Tobias JD. Neonatal pain management. Saudi Arabia Journal of Anaesthesia. 2014;**8**(Suppl 1):S89-S97

[2] Attarian S, Tran LC, Moore A, Stanton G, Meyer E, Moore RP. The neurodevelopmental impact of neonatal morphine administration. Brain Sciences. 2014;**4**:321-334

[3] Riddell RP. Nonpharmacological management of procedural pain in infants and young children: An abridged Cochrane review. Pain Research & Management. 2011;**16**(5):321-330

[4] Effe E, Ozer ZC. Effect of sucrose on pain relief during neonatal immunization injection. Applied Nursing Research. 2007;**20**(1):10-16

[5] Gray L, Watt L, Blass EM. Skin-to-skin contact is analgesic in healthy newborns. Pediatrics. 2000;**105**:e14

[6] Zargham-Boroujeni A, Elsagh A, Mohammadizadeh M. The effects of massage and breastfeeding on response to venipuncture pain among hospitalized neonates. Iranian Journal of Nursing and Midwifery Research 2017;**22**(4):308-312

[7] Tiffany Field. Touch for socioemotional and physical well-being: A review. Developmental Review. 2010;**30**:367-383

Chapter 8

Prevention of Procedural Pain in Neonates

Dulce Cruz

Abstract

Neonates admitted to neonatal intensive care units are exposed to a high number of painful procedures for their survival. Faced with a pain that is predictable, it is imperative to implement analgesia before carrying out the procedure, to reduce the impact of the painful experience, maximize the infant's capacity for recovery, and activate their internal inhibitory control system. In addition, other sources of stress are present in an intensive care environment, which contribute to increase sensitivity of the neonates to future episodes of pain. To minimize the consequences of this harmful environment, especially in the most vulnerable babies, premature and/or those with a serious clinical situation, there are validated recommendations for special care to wherever possible prevent pain, family's empowerment for comfort care, and support. Pain management is not just about administering a medication or another treatment, but rather integrated approaches that reduce or block the nociceptive activity of the trauma associated with invasive procedures. To minimize the adverse effects, pain management in neonatal care units requires the use of effective pharmacological and non-pharmacological interventions. The selection of analgesic interventions by healthcare professionals will depend on the type of the procedure, as well as the clinical condition of the newborn.

Keywords: neonate pain, painful procedures, procedural pain, prevention of pain, pain management

1. Introduction

Neonates in need of special care are exposed to high levels of stress and pain. The International Association for the Study of Pain considers pain as an unpleasant sensory and emotional experience associated with actual or potential tissue damage, or as described in terms of such harm [1]. In neonatal care units, pain from medical procedures for diagnosis or treatment purposes falls under this definition.

Around 24 weeks of gestation, pain pathways are already present, with the ability to detect and transmit sensory information about pain events. Although babies do not verbalize their pain, it is not impossible for them to feel and experience it [2].

Several studies demonstrate the impact of unrelieved pain in early childhood, on the clinical stability of neonates and on the potential to change the physiology of their developing nervous system, on their sensitivity to behavioral abnormalities later in life. To minimize hyperalgesia and allodynia, especially in the most vulnerable infants with severe sickness, the reduction of adverse environment is recommended [3, 4].

For good practices and the safety of neonates in healthcare environments, professionals must consider that if a medical procedure is painful for adults, it will be also painful for infants. This chapter will focus on painful procedures performed on neonates, except pain following surgery, chronic pain, or other painful stimulus persistent in time (e.g., mechanical ventilation).

Some neonates are at high risk of suffering undertreatment of pain, efforts should be focused on those procedures most frequently and on more vulnerable neonates. The key to minimize expected pain in the context of neonate care is the anticipation of the analgesia. There are effective pharmacological and non-pharmacological interventions for pain management. Despite the existence of guidelines for the prevention and minimization of pain associated with invasive procedures, the incorporation of evidence into clinical practice tends to be slow or incomplete. According to studies there is a higher frequency of painful procedures performed in very preterm babies and on those which have a high severity of the disease. For every day of hospitalization, researchers have observed 5 to 17 painful procedures in neonates. Preprocedural analgesia according to guidelines is an actual and a current concern, there is a high variability of practices between clinicians and units of care [5, 6].

2. Pain in neonates

Painful stimulus performed in neonates activates their sympathetic nervous system, which is observable by physiologic changes such as the increase of the heart rate, intracranial pressure, and blood pressure, as by the decrease of the oxygen saturation. Additional observable effects could be included, such as respiratory patterns, sweating, and skin color changes. During painful stimulation, there are also observed behaviourally changes in neonate facial expression, bodily movement, changes in sleeping, activity level, restlessness, and crying. The facial expression of an infant in pain is characterized by an open mouth, bulging brow, eyes squeezed tight shut, taut cupped tongue, and a deepening of the furrow between the nose and corner of the mouth.

When infants are not provided with pain relief, they become stressed, and their cortisol levels increase. Electroencephalography or electromyography methods have been used to identify pain in infants which are useful for the research of the efficacy of several measures for pain management.

Assessing pain is fundamental for making good clinical decisions, must be undertaken, and documented in the individual process of care of the neonate. In this context, pain assessment should be done before, during, and after each potentially painful intervention to evaluate the efficacy of the pre-emptive analgesia, as on the recovery of the neonate to physiological and behavioral changes.

The tools most widely used and recommended for acute pain and clinical practice are summarized in **Table 1** [6, 7].

Assessment tool	Population	Physiologic indicators	Behavioral indicators	Context	Score
NFCS *Neonatal Facial Coding Scale* [8]	Preterm and term neonates, infants at 4 months of age	None	Facial muscle group movement		0–10
PIPP Premature Infant Pain Profile revised [9]	Preterm and term newborn <28 weeks	Heart rate Oxygen saturation	Facial expression	Gestational age Alert status	Full-term newborn 0–18 Preterm newborn 0–21
NIPS Neonatal Infant Pain Scale [10]	Preterm and term newborn 28–41 weeks	Breathing pattern	Facial expression Crying Movements of the upper and lower limbs	Alert status	0–7
BPSN Bernese Pain Scale for Neonates [11]	Preterm and term newborn 27–41 weeks	Breathing pattern Heart rate Oxygen saturation Skin color	Duration of crying Time to calm down. Facial expression Posture	Alert status	0–27
NIAPAS Neonatal Infant Acute Pain Assessment Scale [12]	Preterm and term newborn 23–42 weeks	Heart rate Oxygen saturation Breathing pattern	Facial expression Crying Muscle tone Reaction to manipulation	Gestational age Alert status	0–18
N-PASS Neonatal Pain, Agitation, and Sedation Scale [13]	Preterm and term newborn 23–40 weeks	Vital signs	Crying Facial expression Muscle tone	Gestational age Alert status	Pain 0 a 10 Sedation −10 a 0
EDIN Echelle Douleur Inconfort Nouveau-né [14]	Preterm newborn 25–36 weeks	None	Facial expression Body Movements Quality of interaction Comfort	Sleep quality	0 a 15

Table 1.
Acute pain assessment tools on neonates.

3. Predictability of pain on neonatal interventions

Painful events performed in neonatal care units are associated with actual or potential tissue damage of the skin or mucosae of the neonates. According to the degree of the invasiveness of the procedure, it should be categorized as mild to severe pain predictability (**Table 2**) [7–15].

Pain scores[a]	Mild (0–3)	Moderate (4–6)	Severe (7–10)
Painful procedures	Feeding tube placement Nasal, Oral suctioning Umbilical catheterization Urinary catheter insertion Gastric tube insertion Adhesive removal	Heelstick[b] Intramuscular injection[b] Subcutaneous injection[b] Venipuncture[b] Intravenous cannulation[b] Drain removal Peripheral insertion of central catheter[b] Tracheal aspiration Wound treatment	Tracheal intubation Chest-drain insertion[b] Lumbar puncture[b] Eye treatment for retinopathy of prematurity

[a]*According to Neonatal Facial Coding Scale.*
[b]*Needle procedure.*

Table 2.
Categorization of painful procedures performed in neonates.

4. Procedural pain management

All neonates have the right to receive optimal comfort to minimize stress and pain, supported by healthcare professionals and their parents. As expected that care providers prevent or treat any infant experiencing pain, avoiding unnecessary pain and discomfort, using appropriate non-pharmacological and pharmacological interventions.

In a neonatal context it is preconized to minimize the impact of the painful experience, with a focus on the maximization of the ability of neonates to recover from it. In this sense, it is not just administering a drug or another treatment, but performing an integrated approach that reduces or blocks the nociceptive activity of the trauma associated with the painful procedure and modifies the situational factors that aggravate it.

The key to manage the pain of invasive procedures is its anticipation. A variety of non-pharmacologic strategies can be implemented in conjunction with pharmacological interventions. Parents or caregivers should be involved to help with comfort measures of pain relief.

Taking care of the environment should be added to the pre-emptive analgesia for painful procedures (**Table 3**). Minimization of acoustic, visual, tactile, or vestibular stimuli, safeguarding sleep, protecting skin, and optimizing nutrition, reduces stress, and increases the comfort and stability of the neonates [15, 16].

4.1 Non-pharmacologic interventions

The quality of procedural pain management in neonates should include neuroprotective core measures, and follow the family-centred care (e.g., partnering with families, and positioning) [7–15].

4.1.1 Positioning, containment, and swaddling

These interventions consist of restricting the movement of the limbs, and limiting the proprioceptive activity of the tactile system of the newborn. In the neonatal context, containment promotes self-regulation and is not exclusive to the performance of painful procedures but is also considered a protective developmental care measure. As a non-pharmacological intervention, it is recommended to start 3 minutes before,

Environmental measures
• Promoting silence; minimize the sound of the monitoring devices in the unit.
• Promoting sleep and rest.
• Promoting day-night cycle.
• Protection from bright light, either using dimmable spotlights or using covers in the incubators.
Behavioral measures
• Minimal manipulation of the neonate.
• Reduction in the number of procedures (e.g., grouping laboratory tests), and selection of the less painful method (e.g., venepuncture versus heel lance for blood collection).
• Performed painful procedures only when justified (e.g., aspiration of secretions)
• Protect skin, use the minimum number of adhesives, and remove it carefully.
• Preparatory information and parental involvement regarding pain management strategies (e.g., physical contact).
• Containment of the newborn.
Optimal analgesia prior to invasive procedures
• Non-pharmacological interventions
• Pharmacological interventions

Table 3.
Beneficial measures to protect neonates.

and remain during and after the procedure until recovery of the neonate. Studies have shown that swaddling a preterm reduces the pulse rate in response to procedural pain.

For all procedures consider these strategies, but with considering the association of others non-pharmacological or pharmacological interventions depending on the degree of the pain of the procedure.

4.1.2 Sweet solutions and breastfeeding

Sweet solutions are recommended by numerous professional organizations; however, inconsistencies are raised regarding their classification, especially in relation to sucrose, categorized as a non-pharmacological, or pharmacological intervention. In this chapter, sweet solutions are considered and included in the non-pharmacological group.

Administration of sucrose (24%), glucose (20 to 30%), or breast milk, alone or in combination with other interventions, has been widely studied for the relief of acute pain in preterm and full-term neonates.

Many protocols recommend giving a sweet solution 2 minutes prior to the painful procedure with an estimated volume of 0.5 to 2.0 ml, administered in the anterior portion of the tongue. The recommended dose for a full-term neonate is approximately 2 ml, for premature infants the dose will be smaller (4–10 ml is the total volume of sucrose that can be administered in a 24-hour period).

Breastfeeding, when available, should be the first choice to relieve pain when undergoing painful procedures, such as venepuncture or during heel lance for blood collection. It consists of placing the newborn on the breast, before, during, and after the procedure, and should not be discontinued.

Breastfeeding significantly decreases the variability of the physiological responses of the newborn compared with other interventions (e.g., containment, non-nutritive sucking, and/or administration of sucrose). There is a smaller increase in heart rate, a decrease in the duration of total crying time, and pain intensity. Breastfeeding is a natural alternative and has a similar efficacy to other sweet solutions. In the unavailability of breastfeeding for reasons associated with the mother or the newborn clinical conditions, only breast milk can be used; however, the associated multisensory experience is lost, and analgesic efficacy is lower.

4.1.3 Pacifier and non-nutritive sucking

Non-nutritive sucking refers to the use of a pacifier to promote infant sucking.

The sucking behavior begins to be present between the 24th and 27th week of gestation; however, it's from the 34th week that becomes rhythmic and strong. Pacifier provides a pain-relieving effect by decreasing the baby's vitality level and crying time. Studies have suggested that sucking triggers the secretion of serotonin, which directly or indirectly affects the transmission of painful stimuli.

It is recommended to associate non-nutritive sucking with containment, kangaroo care, and/or administration of sweet solutions, including breast milk. Some issues associated with this intervention require special attention in the Baby Friendly Hospital Program where the use of pacifiers is only allowed for newborns in the context of procedural pain management.

4.1.4 Kangaroo care

Kangaroo care has become an accepted practice in many neonatal care units and has been found to be effective in minimizing preterm infants' pain response to heel sticks. The combination of being with body skin-to-skin contact and hearing a familiar voice helps neonates to regulate themselves. The Kangaroo care method is a natural measure, economic, increasing the release of endorphins in painful stimuli in newborn babies, and is effective in maintaining parents-baby attachment to reduce pain during invasive procedures. Skin-to-skin contact requires time of preparation, and it's necessary to implement 15 minutes early of the painful procedure.

Low birth weight, neonates weighing <2000 g who are clinically stable should be provided Kangaroo Care early in the first week of life.

4.2 Pharmacological interventions

Pharmacological methods are often needed to control severe acute pain. Although there is significant advances in this area, the balance between pain relief and the risk-benefit of drug effects for neonates remains a challenge for healthcare teams.

Pharmacological options have been investigated in clinical trials with infants, widely tested, and implemented for analgesia on procedural pain.

The most used for moderate-to-severe pain are acetaminophen and the nonsteroidal anti-inflammatory drug, in combination with opioids (e.g., morphine, fentanyl), or adjuvant analgesics namely sedatives, antidepressants, or anticonvulsants.

Nowadays there are other options, such as local anesthetic cream (effective only after 30 to 60 minutes of application, depending on the specific medication), or appropriate analgesia administered by a non-painful route, such as intranasal fentanyl.

The following table briefly presents analgesia recommendations for the most frequent procedures performed in neonatal units of care (**Table 4**) [7–15].

Procedure	Analgesia	Recommendations
Gastric tube insertion	Non-pharmacological measures.	Perform rapidly, and avoid injury. Use lubricant.
Umbilical catheterization	Non-pharmacological measures.	Avoid sutures on skin around the umbilical stump
Tracheal aspiration in ventilated newborn	Non-pharmacological measures. Consider opioid infusion.	Consider this procedure only when secretions are present and not routinely. Perform the technique rapidly, preferably in a closed circuit, with 4 hands. Limit aspiration to the beginning of the endotracheal tube.
Venipuncture Intravenous cannulation	Non-pharmacological measures. Consider topical anesthetic.	
Heelstick	Non-pharmacological measures. Consider skin-to-skin contact.	Venipuncture should be considered. Gentle manipulation of the heel. Use mechanical devices instead of the manual lance. Note: Topical anesthetic, acetaminophen, and warming heel are ineffective.
Peripheral insertion of central catheter	Non-pharmacological measures. Consider topical anesthetic. Consider opioid infusion.	
Subcutaneous and intramuscular injections	Non-pharmacological measures. Consider topical anesthetic.	Avoid the intramuscular route, preferring, whenever possible, the intravenous route.
Suprapubic puncture	Non-pharmacological measures Topical anesthetic Consider acetaminophen, opioid infusion, or subcutaneous infiltration—nerve block	
Tracheal intubation	Consider opioid infusion, a small dose of intravenous ketamine. Intubation with a muscle relaxant (if an experienced clinician is present) is strongly recommended.	Intubation without analgesia only in delivery room resuscitation situations and/or emergency situations. Ideal sequence: 1. Oxygen 2. Neuromuscular blocking agents 3. Analgesic and/or hypnotic 4. Muscle relaxant
Wound dressing	Non-pharmacological measures. Consider acetaminophen, and opioid infusion.	Consider acetaminophen, opioid infusion, *deep sedation, or general anesthesia for extensive or deep wounds.*
Ophthalmological screening	Non-pharmacological measures. Consider topical anesthetic (eye drops). Consider opioid infusion with opioid bolus or ketamine.	Avoid or use blepharostat instruments. Monitor the procedure with the appropriate pain scale.
Chest tube removal	Non-pharmacological measures. Consider topical anesthetic.	

Procedure	Analgesia	Recommendations
Chest tube placement	Non-pharmacological measures. Topical anesthetic. Consider opioid infusion.	Opioid bolus in ventilated neonates. In non-ventilated patients, consider ketamine bolus, always anticipating the need for ventilatory support. Monitor procedure with appropriate pain tools and adjust analgesia (bolus or opioid perfusion) according to the score of pain.
Lumbar puncture	Non-pharmacological measures. Consider topical anesthetic if not urgent or subcutaneous infiltration with lidocaine. Consider opioid infusion or midazolam.	Avoid extreme flexion of the neck, regardless of the selected position (risk of trauma and hypoxemia).

Table 4.
Pain management for the most common neonatal procedures.

The selection of the interventions above described should not be generalized to all neonates but should recognize and follow an individual pain management approach [16]. In all the situations, combining two or more non-pharmacological interventions has an additive and/or synergistic effect on minimizing pain. With pharmacological measures, this association has benefits to reduce the dose, frequency, and possible side effects of the drugs.

Advances in technologies are becoming an opportunity for pain management by healthcare teams, new alert items, pain assessment tools in informatic devices, and new fields for non-pharmacological intervention documentation [17].

5. Recognizing neonates at high risk of pain

The identification of the main factors associated with neonatal procedural pain, allows a better care for pain prevention and protection of premature and/or sick babies in neonatal intensive care units.

Several observational studies identified factors related to a higher incidence of painful procedures in premature infants and in the first 3 days of the neonate in the unit stay [5, 6]. The most frequent acute pain results from skin-breaking procedures. Preterm infants with very low birth weight, and/or neonates receiving nasal oxygen, continuous positive airway pressure, or ventilation support, are exposed to a high number of procedures.

Prematurity is associated with a greater use of specific pre-procedural analgesia, and ventilated preterm neonates, with the lowest gestational age, which has the lowest amount of pharmacological pain relief during procedures. Neonates at the highest risk for neurological impairment have the lowest number of opioids administered during the first day of life.

Sweet-taste solutions are less likely to be used in infants in the first week of life and vary significantly during tissue damaging procedures. Less pre-procedural analgesia is used during the first day of admission as well as during the night shift. Considering the type of painful procedures, pharmacological analgesia is significantly higher for needle sticks.

Regarding organizational context as a predictor for pain management, the existence of pain protocols was not a predictor for analgesia use. Parental presence during procedures was predictive for a greater use of specific pre-procedural analgesia.

Optimal pain management according to clinical guidelines needs to be incremented, especially for procedures with an expected moderate to high score of severe pain, in the first week of a neonate's hospitalization [6].

6. Best practices on procedural pain management

Good practice recommendations are considered essential for clarifying and contextualizing measures to reduce pain associated with painful procedures in neonate care units.

6.1 Preventing neonate pain and relief

- It must be mandatory to anticipate pain before carrying out the procedures.

- Consistent pain management is important to reduce adverse effects, promote comfort, attachment, and self-regulation.

- Consider a multimodal analgesic approach to procedural pain management in neonates.

- Implement effective pain management strategies.

- Family is encouraged, empowered, and supported to provide comfort to their infant.

- The selection of the most appropriate medication-based treatment approach for a preterm or term infant involves a careful analysis of risks and benefits.

- Use the most efficacious and least invasive way to administer analgesic drugs.

- Efforts should be aggregated for the implementation of strategies on modifiable predictive factors for neonates' pain in their first days of life.

- *Developing best-approach protocols* for acute pain in neonates to develop uniformity in pain management and reduce the wide variability of practices.

- Protocols must be updated and multidisciplinary as a clinical tool to support informed decisions about effective pain relief.

- Using standardized pain assessment tools.

- Pain assessment requires training and education.

6.2 Creating a neonate-centred care

- Develop a neonate plan for pain management. Identifying neonates at high risk for painful procedures is essential for optimizing pain care (e.g., critically ill infants, and premature babies).

- Taking a history of the pain, including the history of painful procedures, from the first day of hospitalization of the neonate in the unit. Frequency, location, and intensity, what interventions have been undertaken, and the impact of the pain.

- Observing how the neonate's pain presents, physically, emotionally, and behaviourally. The best way of judging whether a baby is in pain is to observe carefully, and know his patterns.

- Pain assessment should be ongoing and incorporated into the plan of care for all neonates.

- Infant response to analgesic interventions should be documented and guide future management strategies.

- *Empowering the parents*, providing individualized support and family collaboration.

- Providing information to families on the importance of pain management and their involvement in the process.

- Parents were invited to participate in their baby's comfort care.

- Both clinicians and families can work towards the direction of more personalized pain management strategies. For neonates include breastfeeding, non-nutritive sucking, swaddling, skin-to-skin touch, positioning, and containment.

- Parents were permitted to be present at all procedures and to participate in making decisions.

6.3 Decreasing procedural pain

- Routine procedures should be avoided.

- Carry out diagnostic and therapeutic procedures more safely, with materials suitable and with experienced professionals or skills training.

- In relation to more invasive and severe painful procedures, it is suggested to carry out pain management education and multidisciplinary simulation training.

- *Institutionalizing Pain Management.* Appropriate pain management becomes part of the culture of care.

- Creating an interdisciplinary work group with administrative authority to guide changes.
- Development of explicit policies and protocols.
- Create a culture of comfort and reduce pain for all children in the institutional system.
- An ongoing education. Educational initiatives at the site of care in small groups and be repeated frequently.
- Audits with feedback
- Applies to children's rights, 'right to receive relief from pain and suffering to the maximum extent possible'.
- Inadequate pain relief is considered malpractice.

7. Conclusion

Pain is commonly from medical procedures for diagnosis or treatment purposes, performed in newborn infants, term, or preterm, which require special care. To reduce the impact of pain in neonatal units, it is mandatory to associate painful procedures, with effective measures for the prevention of pain. Healthcare professionals and parents recognize the vantages of the implementation of an individualized developmental care approach to reduce and avoid pain and discomfort experienced during neonate stay in the hospital.

Pain is regarded as a human rights issue, and education and skills training are mandatory to perform procedures more safely, with appropriate materials, and optimal pain relief measures. Protocols should be up to date, with a multidisciplinary focus, avoiding unnecessary pain and discomfort in neonates.

Acknowledgements

The author thanks to the Pain in Child Health, a research training initiative of the Canadian Institutes of Health Research, for sharing knowledge and promoting the development of the study of pain in neonates and children. This work is funded by national funds through the Foundation for Science and Technology, under the project UIDP/04923/2020.

Conflict of interest

The authors declare no conflict of interest.

Author details

Dulce Cruz
Nursing Department, University of Évora, Évora, Portugal

*Address all correspondence to: dcruz@uevora.pt

References

[1] Pain terms: A list with definitions and notes on usage. Recommended by the IASP Subcommittee on Taxonomy. Pain. Jun 1979;**6**(3):249. PMID: 460932

[2] Fitzgerald M. The development of nociceptive circuits. Nature reviews. Neuroscience. 2005;**6**(7):507-520. DOI: 10.1038/nrn1701

[3] Walker SM. Biological and neurodevelopmental implications of neonatal pain. Clinics in Perinatology. 2013;**40**(3):471-491. DOI: 10.1016/j.clp.2013.05.002

[4] Brummelte S, Chau C, Cepeda M, Ivan L, Degenhardt A, Weinberg J, et al. Cortisol levels in former preterm children at school age are predicted by neonatal procedural pain-related stress. Psychoneuroendocrinology. 2015;**51**:151-163. DOI: 10.1016/j.psyneuen.2014.09.018

[5] Cruz MD, Fernandes AM, Oliveira C. Epidemiology of painful procedures performed in neonates: A systematic review of observational studies. European Journal of Pain (London, England). 2016;**20**(4):489-498. DOI: 10.1002/ejp.757

[6] Cruz MD. Epidemiologia da dor neonatal [thesis]. Coimbra: Faculty of Medicine, University of Coimbra, Portugal; 2020

[7] Anand KJS. International evidence-based Group for Neonatal Pain. Consensus statement for the prevention and management of pain in the newborn. Archives of pediatric. Adolescent Medicine. 2001;**155**:173-180

[8] Grunau RVE, Craig KD. Pain expression in neonates: Facial action and cry. Pain. 1987;**28**:395-410

[9] Stevens BJ, Gibbins S, Yamada J, Dionne K, Lee G, Johnston C. The premature infant pain profile-revised (PIPP-R): Initial validation and feasibility. Clinical Journal Pain. 2014;**30**:238-243

[10] Lawrence J, Alcock D, McGrath P. The development of a tool to assess neonatal pain. Neonatal Net. 1993;**12**:59-66

[11] Cignacco E, Mueller R, Harmers JP, Gessler P. Pain assessment in the neonate using the Bernese pain scale for neonates. Early Human Development. 2004;**78**:125-131

[12] Pölkki T et al. Development and preliminary validation of the neonatal infant acute pain assessment scale (NIAPAS). International Journal of Nursing Studies. 2014;**51**(12):1585-1594

[13] Hummel P, Puchalski M, Creech SD, Weiss MG. Clinical reliability and validity of the N-PASS: Neonatal pain, agitation and sedation scale with prolonged pain. Journal of Perinatology. 2008;**28**(1):55-60

[14] Debillon T, Zupan V, Ravault N, Magny JF, Dehan M. Development and initial validation of the EDIN scale, a new tool for assessing pro- longed pain in preterm infants. Archives of Disease in Childhood—Fetal and Neonatal Edition. 2001;**85**:F36-F41

[15] Anand KJS. Prevention and Treatment of Neonatal Pain. In: In: Connor RF, editor. UpToDate. Wolters Kluwer; 2023 [Accessed: September 4, 2023]

[16] Coughlin M. Transformative Nursing in the NICU: Trauma-Informed

Age-Appropriate Care. Springer Publishing Company; 2014. pp. 1-199. DOI: 10.1891/9780826196583. ISSN: 0279-5442

[17] EFCNI, Oude-Reimer M, Frauenfelder O, et al. Support during Painful Procedures and Pain Assessment. European Standards of Care for Newborn Health; 2018. pp. 1-62. Available from: https://newborn-health-standards.org/wp-content/uploads/2022/08/2022_09_01_TEG_Care-procedures_all.pdf

Chapter 9

Medication Safety in Neonatal Care

Hossam A. Elgnainy

Abstract

Medication safety is crucial in neonatal care, given neonates' unique vulnerabilities, especially premature infants. This chapter highlights the need for safe medication administration in neonatal settings, given neonates' fragile physiology and susceptibility to errors. It offers an overview of medication safety principles, focusing on equipping healthcare professionals with the knowledge and tools needed for neonatal medication administration. Key areas covered include the medication administration process, with attention to accurate dosing, weight-based calculations, and personalized treatment. Proper medication storage, labeling, and adherence to expiration dates are emphasized. High-risk medications and strategies for risk mitigation are discussed, along with the role of technology in enhancing safety. The chapter also stresses reporting and learning from medication errors, promoting robust reporting systems, blame-free environments, and education for medication safety. In summary, this chapter provides foundational insights for healthcare professionals into neonatal care, enabling safer medication use and improved patient care.

Keywords: adverse drug reactions, dosage calculations, evidence-based practices, high-risk medications, medication administration practices, medication administration routes, medication errors, medication reconciliation, medication safety audits and assessments, medication safety culture, medication safety guidelines, medication safety training and education, neonatal drug formulations, neonatal medication errors reporting, neonatal medication safety, neonatal pharmacokinetics, patient safety in neonatal care, technology and medication safety, medication storage and labeling

1. Introduction

The safe and effective administration of medication to neonates is crucial in neonatal care. Neonates, especially premature infants, require specialized approaches to medication administration due to their unique physiological characteristics and developmental considerations. Understanding and ensuring medication safety in neonatal care involves recognizing the specific challenges and potential risks associated with medication use in this vulnerable population.

This chapter serves as an introduction to medication safety in neonatal care, providing healthcare professionals with valuable insights, principles, practices, and strategies to optimize medication safety for neonates. By addressing key concepts and considerations, we aim to equip healthcare professionals with the necessary knowledge and tools to navigate the complexities of medication administration in neonatal settings.

Neonates are highly susceptible to medication errors and adverse drug events due to their fragile physiology, immature organ systems, and limited ability to metabolize and eliminate medications. Prioritizing medication safety is essential to minimize harm, adverse effects, prolonged hospitalization, and mortality.

The chapter will explore various aspects of medication safety in neonatal care, including medication administration processes such as prescribing, dispensing, preparing, and administering medications. Attention will be given to challenges associated with accurate dosing, weight-based calculations, and individualized dosing regimens to ensure appropriate medication therapy for neonatal patients.

Proper medication storage, labeling, and expiration dates are critical to prevent medication errors and maintain medication efficacy. Medication reconciliation, safety considerations for different routes of medication administration (oral, intravenous, and respiratory), dosage calculations, and compounding in neonatal care will also be discussed.

High-risk medications commonly used in neonatal care will be addressed, along with strategies to mitigate associated risks through monitoring, dose adjustments, and administration techniques. The role of technology and automation in enhancing medication safety, including barcode scanning, smart infusion pumps, and computerized provider order entry (CPOE) systems, will be explored.

Reporting and learning from medication errors will be emphasized, promoting robust reporting systems, blame-free environments, and the use of error reporting data to identify areas for improvement and implement targeted interventions. Education, ongoing training, and competency assessment will be discussed to enhance medication safety awareness and promote best practices among healthcare providers.

By covering these key topics, this chapter aims to provide a solid foundation for healthcare professionals in understanding and implementing medication safety strategies in neonatal care. Through evidence-based practices, practical recommendations, and an interdisciplinary approach, we can strive for safer medication use, minimize errors, and improve the quality of care provided to neonates.

2. Medication administration processes in neonatal care

The administration of medications in neonatal care is a complex and critical process that requires utmost attention to detail and adherence to established protocols. Neonates, especially premature, have unique physiological characteristics and developmental considerations that necessitate specialized approaches to medication administration. Understanding and implementing safe medication administration processes are essential to ensure optimal patient outcomes and minimize the risk of medication errors in this vulnerable population [1].

This section will delve into the various components of medication administration in neonatal care, including prescribing, dispensing, preparing, and administering medications. Each step in the medication administration process presents its own challenges and considerations, requiring healthcare professionals to be knowledgeable, competent, and vigilant.

Prescribing medications for neonates involves careful consideration of factors such as gestational age, weight, organ maturity, and specific indications. Neonatal drug dosing requires meticulous attention to ensure accurate and individualized therapy. Healthcare providers must have a thorough understanding of pharmacokinetics and pharmacodynamics in neonates to determine appropriate dosages and the frequency of administration [2].

To facilitate accurate and safe medication administration, healthcare professionals must have access to reliable and up-to-date drug references and formularies specific to neonatal care. These resources provide essential information on medication compatibility, dosing guidelines, potential drug interactions, and adverse effects. Establishing standardized protocols and clinical guidelines for neonatal medication prescribing promotes consistency and enhances safety across healthcare settings [2].

The dispensing phase involves the procurement and preparation of medications for administration. Pharmacy services play a crucial role in ensuring accurate medication dispensing, including proper labeling, verifying medication orders, and employing quality control measures. The use of barcoding technology in medication dispensing helps reduce errors by ensuring accurate medication identification and verification.

Once the medication is dispensed, healthcare professionals must properly prepare it for administration. This process may involve dilution, reconstitution, or compounding, depending on the medication's form and route of administration. Neonatal medication preparation requires precision and adherence to aseptic techniques to prevent contamination and maintain medication integrity. Healthcare professionals should receive training on proper medication preparation procedures, including accurate measurement, calculation, and mixing techniques [3].

Administering medications to neonates requires meticulous attention to detail and a focus on patient safety. Healthcare providers must consider factors such as the appropriate route of administration, proper technique, and patient comfort. Common routes of medication administration in neonates include oral, intravenous, subcutaneous, and inhalation routes [2, 3].

When administering medications orally, healthcare professionals must consider the infant's ability to swallow and the potential for medication interactions with enteral feeds. The use of oral syringes or specialized devices may be necessary to ensure accurate dosing and minimize the risk of aspiration [1].

Intravenous medication administration in neonates demands precision and expertise. Healthcare providers must carefully calculate and dilute medications to avoid over- or under-dosage. The use of infusion pumps and smart technology can enhance safety by providing accurate infusion rates and monitoring [1, 4].

Subcutaneous medication administration requires knowledge of proper injection techniques, needle size selection, and anatomical considerations in neonates. Ensuring proper rotation of injection sites helps prevent tissue damage and discomfort.

Inhalation medications, such as bronchodilators or surfactants, are commonly used in neonatal care. Healthcare professionals must be proficient in the use of nebulizers, inhalation chambers, or respiratory support devices to deliver medications effectively to the neonatal airway.

Throughout the medication administration process, accurate documentation is essential. Healthcare providers should document medication administration details, including the medication name, dose, route, time of administration, and any observed effects or adverse reactions. Proper documentation supports continuity of care, facilitates communication among healthcare providers, and provides valuable information for medication reconciliation and evaluation [1].

To ensure safe medication administration in neonatal care, interdisciplinary collaboration is crucial. Neonatologists, pediatric pharmacists, nurses, and other healthcare professionals must work together to establish standardized medication administration protocols, provide ongoing education and training, and foster a culture of safety [2].

Medication administration in neonatal care is a multifaceted process that requires meticulous attention to detail, adherence to established protocols, and a comprehensive understanding of neonatal pharmacotherapy. Healthcare professionals involved in medication administration must possess the knowledge, skills, and resources necessary to ensure safe and effective medication use. By implementing evidence-based practices and promoting interdisciplinary collaboration, we can enhance medication safety, improve patient outcomes, and provide optimal care to neonates in need [2].

3. Medication storage, labeling, and expiration dates in neonatal care

Proper medication storage, labeling, and management of expiration dates are critical aspects of ensuring medication safety in neonatal care settings. Neonates, particularly premature, are highly sensitive to the quality and potency of medications, making it essential to implement specific guidelines for medication storage and handling. This section will discuss the importance of appropriate medication storage conditions, accurate labeling practices, and strategies for managing expiration dates in the neonatal population [2].

Medication storage plays a crucial role in maintaining the integrity and stability of medications. Factors such as temperature, humidity, light exposure, and air quality can significantly impact the efficacy and safety of pharmaceutical products. In neonatal care, where even small deviations from recommended storage conditions can have profound effects, it is paramount to establish appropriate storage guidelines [2].

Temperature control is of the utmost importance when storing medications for neonates. Most medications require storage within a specific temperature range, typically between 2°C and 8°C (36°F and 46°F) for refrigerated items and between 15°C and 30°C (59°F and 86°F) for room temperature products. Special attention should be given to medications that are particularly temperature-sensitive, such as certain antibiotics, biologics, and intravenous solutions. Refrigerators used for medication storage should have temperature monitoring systems in place, with regular calibration and documentation of temperature readings.

Humidity control is also vital in medication storage, as excessive humidity can lead to degradation and loss of potency. Neonatal care units should have humidity control measures in place, such as dehumidifiers or moisture-absorbing packets, to maintain an optimal storage environment.

Light exposure can degrade medications, particularly those in light-sensitive containers or packaging. UV-protective measures, such as amber-colored vials or light-blocking storage cabinets, should be utilized to minimize light exposure and preserve medication stability.

Proper labeling of medications is essential for accurate identification, ensuring the correct medication is administered to the neonate. Each medication container should be clearly labeled with the drug name, strength, dosage form, and any specific instructions for use. For compounded medications, additional information, such as the date of preparation, expiration date, and storage conditions, should be included. Labeling should be legible, durable, and resistant to fading or smudging. Barcode labels can also be employed to facilitate accurate medication identification and improve the efficiency of medication administration processes [2, 5].

Managing expiration dates is crucial in neonatal care to ensure the use of medications within their indicated potency and safety limits. Medications should never be used past their expiration dates, as their efficacy and stability may be compromised. Implementing a robust system for monitoring and managing medication expiration dates is essential. This includes regular inventory checks, proper rotation of stock, and removal of expired medications from storage areas [6].

Pharmacy departments in neonatal care settings should establish clear protocols for managing expired medications. This may involve proper disposal procedures, adherence to environmental regulations, and documentation of discarded medications. Education and training programs should be provided to healthcare professionals involved in medication management to ensure understanding and compliance with expiration date policies [3].

Regular audits and quality assurance checks are essential to monitor medication storage practices, labeling accuracy, and adherence to expiration date management. These evaluations can help identify areas for improvement, address any deviations from established protocols, and reinforce a culture of medication safety [3].

Proper medication storage, accurate labeling, and effective management of expiration dates are critical components of medication safety in neonatal care. Neonates are particularly vulnerable to medication-related risks, necessitating meticulous attention to these aspects. By implementing stringent guidelines for storage conditions, ensuring accurate labeling practices, and developing robust expiration date management protocols, healthcare professionals can help mitigate medication errors, maintain medication integrity, and provide the best possible care to neonates in need.

4. Medication reconciliation in the neonatal population

Medication reconciliation is a vital process in healthcare that aims to ensure accurate and comprehensive medication information during care transitions. This section will discuss the importance of medication reconciliation specifically in the neonatal population, where medication safety is of the utmost concern. It will explore the challenges unique to neonatal care and provide strategies for implementing effective medication reconciliation processes [2].

Neonates often undergo multiple care transitions, including transfers between healthcare facilities, shifts in healthcare providers, and changes in medication regimens. Each transition introduces the potential for medication discrepancies, including omissions, duplications, dosage errors, or incorrect medication selections. These discrepancies can lead to adverse drug events, compromised patient safety, and suboptimal treatment outcomes. Medication reconciliation serves as a crucial safeguard against these risks [3].

The process of medication reconciliation involves comparing the medications a neonate is currently taking to those that are intended to be prescribed or administered, with the goal of identifying and resolving any discrepancies [1].

Medication reconciliation in the neonatal population presents unique challenges due to factors such as limited communication abilities, complex medication regimens, and variations in medication orders based on gestational age, weight, and clinical condition. To address these challenges, healthcare professionals involved in neonatal care should adopt specific strategies and best practices:

1. Interprofessional collaboration: effective medication reconciliation requires collaboration among various healthcare providers involved in the neonatal care team, including physicians, pharmacists, nurses, and caregivers. Clear communication channels and standardized processes should be established to facilitate accurate medication information exchange.

2. Standardized medication history collection: developing a standardized approach to collecting medication histories for neonates is crucial. This includes obtaining information from multiple reliable sources, such as the mother, caregivers, and previous healthcare providers. Electronic health records and digital tools can help streamline the collection and organization of medication history data [2].

3. Medication list review: careful review of medication lists should be performed during care transitions, with a focus on identifying any discrepancies, such as medication omissions, duplications, or dosage errors. This review should consider factors specific to neonatal care, such as gestational age, weight, and clinical condition, to ensure appropriate medication selection and dosing.

4. Communication and documentation: accurate and timely communication of medication changes and updates is essential to ensure continuity of care. Documentation of medication reconciliation activities, including any identified discrepancies and their resolution, should be documented in the medical record to facilitate communication among healthcare providers [2].

5. Education and empowerment of caregivers: involving and educating caregivers about medication reconciliation processes can enhance medication safety in neonatal care. Caregivers should be encouraged to provide accurate medication information, ask questions, and actively participate in medication-related discussions and decisions [7, 8].

6. Technology integration: the use of technology, such as electronic prescribing systems, barcode scanning, and electronic health records, can greatly facilitate medication reconciliation in neonatal care. These tools can automate medication list creation, provide real-time medication information, and assist in detecting and resolving medication discrepancies [9–11].

Regular evaluation and quality improvement initiatives should be implemented to assess the effectiveness of medication reconciliation processes in neonatal care. This includes monitoring medication discrepancies, tracking adverse drug events, and soliciting feedback from healthcare providers and caregivers.

Medication reconciliation is a critical process in neonatal care to ensure medication safety during care transitions. By adopting interprofessional collaboration, standardized approaches, effective communication, and the integration of technology, healthcare providers can mitigate medication discrepancies and improve patient outcomes in the neonatal population. Through diligent medication reconciliation practices, we can provide the highest level of care to our neonatal patients, reducing the risk of medication-related harm and promoting optimal health.

5. Safety considerations for different routes of medication administration

In neonatal care, various routes of medication administration are utilized to ensure effective and targeted delivery of medications. Each route has its own safety considerations that healthcare professionals must carefully address to minimize the risk of adverse events and optimize medication outcomes. This section will discuss the safety considerations associated with different routes of medication administration in the neonatal population.

5.1 Oral administration

Oral administration is a common route for medication delivery in neonatal care, particularly for non-emergent and enteral medications. However, several safety considerations should be taken into account:

- Swallowing and absorption: neonates may have difficulty swallowing, especially premature neonates. It is important to ensure that the medication is appropriately formulated to facilitate swallowing and absorption. Liquid formulations with the use of oral syringes can enhance medication administration accuracy and minimize the risk of aspiration.

- Dosing accuracy: neonates require precise dosing to avoid underdosing or overdosing. Liquid medications should be measured accurately using calibrated devices, such as oral syringes or droppers. Careful attention should be given to dose calculations based on the neonate's weight, gestational age, and specific medication guidelines.

- Taste and palatability: Medication taste and palatability may affect compliance in neonates. Adding sweeteners or using flavored formulations can improve acceptability. However, it is important to consider any potential interactions between medications and added ingredients [2].

5.2 Intravenous administration

Intravenous (IV) administration allows for rapid drug delivery and immediate onset of action. However, it carries inherent risks and requires careful attention to safety considerations:

- Venous access: establishing and maintaining venous access can be challenging in neonates. The selection of appropriate venous access devices, such as peripheral intravenous catheters or umbilical venous catheters, should consider factors such as catheter size, insertion technique, and catheter dwell time. Proper site care and monitoring for complications, such as infiltration or infection, are crucial.

- Calculating the osmolarity of the medication to be administered and making sure the osmolarity is suitable for the access site is of great importance to avoid side effects such as extravasation. For example, any solution of osmolarity greater than 900 mOsm/L should be administered in a central line and contraindicated with peripheral lines.

- Dilution and compatibility: intravenous medications often require dilution prior to administration. It is essential to ensure proper dilution techniques and compatibility with other medications and fluids to prevent precipitation or adverse reactions. Standardized guidelines and protocols should be followed for safe IV medication preparation and administration.

- Infusion rate and monitoring: neonates have specific fluid and medication requirements. Infusion rates should be carefully calculated and monitored to prevent fluid overload or rapid administration of medications. Continuous monitoring of vital signs, infusion rates, and potential medication-specific adverse effects is essential [12].

5.3 Topical administration

Topical medications, such as creams, ointments, and patches, are commonly used in neonatal care. Safety considerations for topical administration include:

- Skin integrity: neonatal skin is delicate and prone to damage. Careful assessment of skin integrity, particularly in preterm neonates, is necessary before applying topical medications. The selection of appropriate formulations and avoidance of irritants are essential to prevent skin irritation or adverse reactions.

- Absorption and systemic effects: topical medications can be absorbed systemically, especially in premature neonates with immature skin barriers. Healthcare professionals should be aware of the potential for systemic effects, drug interactions, and cumulative effects of repeated applications. Close monitoring of neonates receiving topical medications is important [1].

5.4 Respiratory administration

Respiratory medications, such as inhalers or nebulized treatments, are commonly used in neonates with respiratory conditions. Safety considerations for respiratory administration include:

- Proper technique: healthcare professionals should be skilled in proper inhaler or nebulizer technique to ensure effective medication delivery. Correct device selection, appropriate dosing, and proper instruction to caregivers are crucial.

- Spacer use: the use of spacers or valved holding chambers can improve drug delivery and reduce the risk of side effects. The selection of an appropriate spacer size for neonates and regular cleaning are important considerations.

- Infection prevention: nebulizer equipment should be cleaned and disinfected according to guidelines to prevent cross-contamination and the risk of respiratory infections. Strict infection control measures, including hand hygiene, should be followed during respiratory medication administration [2].

5.5 Parenteral administration

Parenteral routes, such as subcutaneous, intramuscular, or intrathecal injections, are used for specific medications or situations in neonatal care. Safety considerations for parenteral administration include:

- Needle selection and site preparation: neonatal skin is fragile, and needle selection should consider the infant's size and the medication's viscosity. Proper site preparation, adherence to aseptic techniques, and the use of appropriate needle lengths and gauges can minimize the risk of tissue damage or infection.

- Injection technique: healthcare professionals should be skilled in proper injection techniques to ensure accurate and safe administration. Knowledge of specific injection sites, depth, and avoidance of critical structures is important to prevent complications.

- Pain management: neonates experience pain during injections. The use of appropriate pain management strategies, such as local anesthesia, distraction techniques, or non-pharmacological interventions, should be considered to minimize pain and distress.

It is crucial for healthcare professionals to stay updated with evidence-based guidelines and best practices regarding medication administration routes in neonatal care. Regular training, competency assessments, and interprofessional collaboration are essential to ensure safe and effective medication administration in this vulnerable population. By addressing the specific safety considerations for each route, healthcare providers can minimize risks and optimize medication outcomes for neonates [12].

6. Dosage calculations and compounding in neonatal care

Dosage calculations and compounding in neonatal care play a crucial role in ensuring accurate and safe medication administration. Neonates, due to their unique physiological characteristics and variability in drug metabolism, require individualized dosage regimens. Healthcare professionals involved in neonatal care, including pharmacists, nurses, and physicians, must possess the knowledge and skills necessary to perform accurate dosage calculations and compounding. This section will discuss the importance of dosage calculations and compounding in neonatal care and highlight key considerations and best practices [4].

6.1 Dosage calculations

Neonatal dosage calculations involve determining the appropriate dose of a medication based on the infant's weight, gestational age, postnatal age, renal and hepatic function, and other factors. Neonates have a larger drug distribution volume than adults for hydrophilic medications and limited drug distribution volume for lipophilic medications, decreased drug clearance, and immature organ systems, which affect drug pharmacokinetics and pharmacodynamics. As a result, dosage calculations need to be precise to avoid under-dosing or overdosing.

Several methods can be employed to calculate neonatal drug dosages, including body weight-based calculations, body surface area calculations, and dosage adjustment based on gestational age, postnatal age, or both. Healthcare professionals must have a thorough understanding of these calculation methods and the specific considerations for each medication and the route of administration. Additionally, the use of technology, such as specialized neonatal drug dosing calculators or computerized physician order entry systems, can enhance accuracy and efficiency in dosage calculations.

6.2 Example for neonatal dose calculation

If our patient is a 3 kg term neonate and to be given Meropenem 40 mg/kg/8 h, the dose should be calculated as follows:

1. Identify the available Meropenem product:

    - For example, Meropenem 500 mg powder vial, to be reconstituted.

2. Identify the method of preparation according to the monograph, hospital formulary, or product leaflet:

    - Reconstitute the vial of 500 mg powder with 10 ml normal saline.

3. Calculate the concentration of the product:

    - In this example, it will be 50 mg/ml, as 500 mg reconstituted with 10 ml.

4. Calculate the total amount to be given to the patient:

    - In this example, 120 mg/dose, as 3 kg patient prescribed with 40 mg/kg/dose.

5. Calculate the total volume to be given to the patient:

    - As the patient needs 120 mg, and the solution prepared concentration is 50 mg/ml, so the patient will receive 2.4 ml/dose.

6. Identify the recommended final concentration that should be administered to the patient, from the monograph, hospital formulary, or product leaflet:

    - For example, 20 mg/ml, so we need to further dilute the 2.4 ml up to 6 ml.

7. Identify the recommended infusion rate that is appropriate to this patient, from the monograph, hospital formulary, or product leaflet:

    - For example: infuse over 1 hour.

6.3 Compounding

In neonatal care, compounding refers to the preparation of individualized medication formulations or doses to meet the specific needs of neonates. Neonates often require medications in lower doses or in different formulations (e.g., oral suspensions, transdermal gels) that may not be commercially available. Compounding allows healthcare professionals to tailor medications to the unique requirements of neonates, ensuring optimal therapeutic outcomes.

Compounding in neonatal care involves various aspects, including selecting the appropriate dosage form, determining the necessary concentration or strength of the medication, and employing appropriate compounding techniques to ensure accuracy, sterility, and stability. Pharmacists and pharmacy technicians play a vital role in compounding medications for neonates, following established compounding guidelines, quality assurance procedures, and regulatory requirements.

It is essential to consider the potential risks associated with compounding, such as contamination, variability in drug concentration, and stability issues. Therefore, strict adherence to aseptic techniques, compounding guidelines, and quality control measures is crucial to ensure the safety and efficacy of compounded medications for neonates. Additionally, proper documentation and labeling of compounded medications are essential for traceability and accurate administration [1].

6.4 Best practices and safety considerations

To enhance safety in dosage calculations and compounding for neonates, healthcare professionals should adhere to the following best practices:

1. Use standardized references and guidelines: healthcare professionals should consult evidence-based references, such as neonatal drug formularies, therapeutic guidelines, and dosage calculation references specific to neonatal care. These resources provide accurate information on dosing recommendations, drug interactions, and potential adverse effects.

2. Double-check calculations and compounding: double-checking calculations and compounding processes can help identify and prevent errors. Implementing an independent double-check process, involving another qualified healthcare professional, helps ensure accuracy and mitigate the risk of medication errors.

3. Regular education and training: healthcare professionals involved in neonatal care should receive ongoing education and training on dosage calculations and compounding practices. This includes staying updated with the latest evidence, guidelines, and technological advancements in neonatal pharmacotherapy.

4. Quality assurance and documentation: implementing robust quality assurance measures, such as periodic inspections, equipment calibration, and proficiency testing, ensures the integrity and accuracy of compounded medications. Documentation of compounding processes, ingredients used, and expiration dates is essential for traceability and accountability.

5. Collaboration and interprofessional communication: collaboration among healthcare professionals, including pharmacists, nurses, and physicians, is vital in ensuring accurate dosage calculations and compounding. Effective communication and sharing of information regarding medication orders, compounding requirements, and potential safety concerns are critical for patient safety.

6. Adherence to regulatory requirements: compliance with regulatory standards and guidelines governing compounding practices, such as USP <797> or relevant local regulations, is essential. Healthcare facilities should establish policies and procedures that align with these standards and ensure adherence to regulatory requirements.

By following these best practices and safety considerations, healthcare professionals can enhance accuracy, minimize the risk of medication errors, and ensure optimal medication therapy for neonates.

Dosage calculations and compounding are integral components of medication administration in neonatal care. Accurate dosage calculations and appropriate compounding practices are essential for ensuring therapeutic efficacy, minimizing medication errors, and promoting patient safety. Healthcare professionals involved in neonatal care should possess the necessary knowledge, skills, and resources to perform precise dosage calculations and compounding, adhering to best practices and safety guidelines [3, 13].

7. High-risk medications in neonatal care

High-risk medications in neonatal care refer to medications that have a higher potential for adverse effects or medication errors. Due to the vulnerability of neonates and their unique physiological characteristics, special attention must be given when prescribing, preparing, and administering high-risk medications. This section will discuss common high-risk medications in neonatal care and the associated safety measures to mitigate the risks involved [5, 8, 13].

7.1 Intravenous (IV) medications

IV medications are frequently used in neonatal care and carry inherent risks such as medication errors, infusion-related complications, and infections. Safety measures to minimize these risks include [6]:

- Accurate patient identification and verification before administering IV medications.

- Use of standardized protocols for medication dilution, preparation, and administration.

- Careful monitoring of infusion rates, particularly for medications with narrow therapeutic windows.

- Adherence to aseptic techniques during IV-line insertion and maintenance to prevent infections.

- Regular assessment of IV sites for signs of infiltration or extravasation.

7.2 Cardiovascular medications

Medications used to manage cardiovascular conditions in neonates, such as inotropic agents and antiarrhythmics, require close monitoring and precise dosing. Safety measures include:

- Calculation of medication doses based on weight and hemodynamic parameters.
- Continuous cardiac monitoring during medication administration to assess adverse effects or changes in the heart rate and rhythm.
- Regular assessment of vital signs and monitoring for signs of medication toxicity or adverse reactions.
- Adherence to specific administration guidelines, such as slow infusion rates or continuous infusions, as prescribed by the healthcare provider.

7.3 Antibiotics

Neonates are susceptible to infections, and antibiotics are frequently prescribed. However, inappropriate antibiotic use can contribute to the development of antibiotic resistance. Safety measures include:

- Accurate identification of the infecting pathogen through appropriate diagnostic testing, when feasible, to guide antibiotic selection.
- Appropriate dosing based on the neonate's weight, renal function, and gestational age.
- Timely administration of antibiotics, particularly for severe infections.
- Regular monitoring of renal and hepatic function to ensure appropriate dosing adjustments and prevent medication toxicity.
- Promotion of antibiotic stewardship principles, such as avoiding broad-spectrum antibiotics when narrower spectrum options are sufficient.

7.4 Sedatives and analgesics

Neonates may require sedation and analgesia for various medical procedures or management of pain. Safety measures include:

- Accurate assessment of pain levels and appropriate selection of analgesics based on the neonate's gestational age and other factors.
- Close monitoring of sedation levels and vital signs during medication administration.

- Avoidance of medication accumulation or oversedation through appropriate dosing intervals and dose adjustments based on the neonate's response.

- Regular assessment for potential adverse effects, such as respiratory depression or changes in oxygen saturation.

7.5 Parenteral nutrition

Parenteral nutrition, comprising a complex mixture of macronutrients, electrolytes, vitamins and trace elements, is commonly administered to neonates who cannot tolerate enteral feeding. Safety measures include:

- Accurate compounding and preparation of parenteral nutrition solutions, following established guidelines and standards.

- Regular monitoring of fluid and electrolyte balance to ensure appropriate adjustments in parenteral nutrition composition.

- Adherence to aseptic techniques during central line insertion and maintenance to prevent infections.

- Regular assessment of liver function and monitoring for signs of parenteral nutrition-associated liver disease.

7.6 Chemotherapeutic agents

In certain cases, neonates may require chemotherapy for the management of malignancies or other serious conditions. Safety measures include:

- Collaboration among an interprofessional team, including oncologists, pharmacists, and nurses, to ensure appropriate dosing and monitoring of chemotherapy.

- Adherence to established protocols for chemotherapy administration, including proper handling, preparation, and disposal of hazardous drugs.

- Close monitoring of hematological and renal parameters during chemotherapy to assess for potential toxicity.

- Implementation of strategies to minimize the exposure of healthcare professionals to hazardous drugs.

To mitigate the risks associated with high-risk medications, healthcare professionals involved in neonatal care should undergo specialized training, have access to evidence-based guidelines, and adhere to medication safety protocols. Additionally, effective communication among the healthcare team, diligent monitoring, and continuous quality improvement initiatives are essential to ensure the safe and effective use of high-risk medications in neonatal care.

By implementing these safety measures, healthcare professionals can minimize medication errors, enhance patient outcomes, and contribute to the overall quality and safety of neonatal care [3, 14].

8. Technology and automation in enhancing medication safety

Technology and automation play a vital role in enhancing medication safety in neonatal care. With their ability to streamline processes, reduce errors, and improve communication, technological advancements have significantly improved medication management practices. This section will explore the various ways in which technology and automation contribute to medication safety in the neonatal setting [10, 11].

8.1 Electronic health records (EHRs)

EHRs have revolutionized healthcare documentation by providing a centralized platform for storing and accessing patient information. In neonatal care, EHRs facilitate accurate and real-time medication-related data, including medication orders, allergies, and administration records. Benefits of EHRs in medication safety include [11]:

- Improved legibility and reduction of medication errors caused by illegible handwriting.
- Enhanced medication reconciliation by electronically comparing medication orders with the patient's medication history.
- Integration with clinical decision support systems to alert healthcare professionals of potential medication interactions, allergies, or dosing errors.
- Facilitation of communication and information sharing among the healthcare team, ensuring consistent and up-to-date medication information.

8.2 Barcode medication administration (BCMA)

BCMA is a technology that uses barcode scanning to ensure accurate medication administration. Each medication package is labeled with a unique barcode that contains information such as the medication name, dosage, and expiration date. Benefits of BCMA in neonatal care include [11]:

- Verification of medication administration accuracy by matching the barcode on the medication package with the patient's identification band.
- Prevention of medication errors by alerting healthcare professionals if the wrong medication or dose is scanned.
- Real-time documentation of medication administration, ensuring accurate and up-to-date medication records.
- Integration with EHRs to facilitate seamless documentation and reduce manual data entry errors.

8.3 Automated medication dispensing systems

Automated medication dispensing systems, such as medication carts or cabinets, help streamline medication storage and distribution processes. These systems offer the following advantages in neonatal care:

- Secure storage of medications, reducing the risk of unauthorized access or medication mix-ups.

- Barcode scanning and verification of medications before dispensing, ensuring accurate medication selection.

- Automated inventory management, with alerts for low stock or expired medications, reducing the risk of administering outdated or unavailable medications.

- Enhanced tracking of medication usage and auditing capabilities, enabling better control over medication supply and reducing the risk of medication diversion.

8.4 Smart infusion pumps

Smart infusion pumps are programmable devices that deliver intravenous medications or fluids at controlled rates. In neonatal care, smart infusion pumps offer the following safety features [9]:

- Dose error reduction through the use of preprogrammed medication libraries with recommended dosing parameters.

- Integration with EHRs to facilitate automatic infusion rate calculations based on the patient's weight, age, and medication parameters.

- Alarms and alerts for potential infusion-related errors, such as incorrect infusion rates or air infusion.

- Drug library customization to align with neonatal-specific medication dosing guidelines and safety protocols.

8.5 Clinical decision support systems (CDSS)

CDSS provides healthcare professionals with evidence-based recommendations, alerts, and reminders at the point of care. In neonatal care, CDSS can support medication safety by [6]:

- Providing dosing recommendations based on the neonate's weight, gestational age, postnatal age, and renal function, reducing the risk of medication errors.

- Alerting healthcare professionals of potential drug interactions or allergies before medication administration.

- Offering clinical guidelines and protocols for specific neonatal conditions, ensuring standardized and evidence-based medication practices.

- Assisting in the selection of appropriate medications by considering factors such as safety, efficacy, and formulary restrictions.

8.6 Telepharmacy and remote medication verification

Telepharmacy and remote medication verification allow pharmacists to review medication orders and verify their accuracy remotely. Benefits of these technologies in neonatal care include [6]:

- Access to pharmacist expertise and verification services in remote or underserved areas.
- Real-time review of medication orders, ensuring accuracy and adherence to neonatal-specific dosing guidelines.
- Timely resolution of medication-related inquiries or concerns, promoting safe and effective medication use.
- Collaboration with the healthcare team, providing recommendations and guidance for complex medication therapies.

Technology and automation have revolutionized medication safety practices in neonatal care. From electronic health records and barcode medication administration to automated dispensing systems and smart infusion pumps, these advancements have improved accuracy, streamlined processes, and reduced the risk of medication errors. By integrating technology into neonatal care settings and leveraging its benefits, healthcare professionals can enhance medication safety, minimize adverse events, and improve the overall quality of care provided to neonates.

9. Reporting and learning from medication errors

Reporting and learning from medication errors is a crucial aspect of medication safety in neonatal care. Errors can occur despite the best intentions and efforts of healthcare professionals, but it is essential to have systems in place to identify, report, analyze, and learn from these incidents. This section will explore the importance of reporting medication errors, the benefits of a culture of transparency and accountability, and strategies for promoting continuous learning and improvement [1, 13, 14].

9.1 Importance of reporting medication errors

Reporting medication errors is vital for several reasons:

- Identification of system weaknesses and vulnerabilities that contribute to errors.
- Prevention of similar errors in the future by implementing targeted interventions.
- Understanding the root causes and contributing factors to develop effective error prevention strategies.
- Fulfillment of ethical and legal obligations to ensure patient safety and promote transparency.

9.2 Culture of transparency and accountability

Creating a culture that encourages reporting and learning from medication errors is crucial. Key elements of a culture of transparency and accountability include:

- Non-punitive approach: healthcare professionals should feel safe reporting errors without fear of punitive actions. Blaming individuals for errors can discourage reporting and hinder learning.

- Supportive environment: encouraging open communication, active listening, and non-judgmental attitudes promotes reporting and facilitates shared learning.

- Leadership commitment: leaders should demonstrate their commitment to medication safety by actively promoting reporting, providing resources for error analysis, and supporting improvement initiatives.

9.3 Reporting systems

Implementing effective reporting systems is essential to capture medication errors. These systems can include:

- Incident reporting systems: establishing a standardized and confidential reporting process enables healthcare professionals to report errors, near misses, or unsafe conditions.

- Anonymous reporting options: allowing anonymous reporting can encourage healthcare professionals who may be hesitant to report errors openly.

- User-friendly platforms: providing accessible and user-friendly reporting platforms enhances engagement and increases reporting rates.

9.4 Error analysis and investigation

Thorough analysis and investigation of reported errors are critical for understanding their underlying causes and developing preventive strategies. Steps involved in error analysis include:

- Collecting data: gathering information about the error, including the medication involved, the context in which it occurred, and any contributing factors.

- Root cause analysis: identifying the root causes of the error, such as communication breakdowns, system failures, or individual factors.

- Human factors analysis: assessing the role of human factors, such as workload, fatigue, distractions, and training, in the occurrence of errors.

- Identifying contributing factors: examining organizational, environmental, and system-level factors that contributed to the error.

- Generating recommendations: developing actionable recommendations to prevent similar errors, improve processes, and enhance medication safety.

9.5 Learning and improvement

Learning from medication errors involves implementing strategies to prevent their recurrence and improve medication safety. This can include:

- Disseminating lessons learned: sharing the findings of error analyses and investigations with healthcare professionals and relevant stakeholders promotes awareness and facilitates knowledge dissemination.

- Implementing targeted interventions: developing and implementing interventions based on identified system weaknesses and contributing factors help prevent future errors.

- Education and training: providing ongoing education and training programs on medication safety, error prevention strategies, and best practices enhances the knowledge and skills of healthcare professionals.

- Continuous quality improvement: establishing mechanisms for continuous monitoring, auditing, and evaluation of medication safety practices helps identify areas for improvement and track progress over time.

By prioritizing the reporting of medication errors, fostering a culture of transparency and accountability, and implementing robust error analysis and learning processes, healthcare organizations can continuously improve medication safety in neonatal care. Through shared learning, effective interventions, and ongoing quality improvement, the goal of minimizing medication errors and ensuring the best possible outcomes for neonates can be achieved [1, 3, 13].

10. Education and training in medication safety

Education and training in medication safety play a crucial role in equipping healthcare professionals with the knowledge, skills, and competencies necessary to ensure optimal medication practices in neonatal care. This section will explore the importance of education and training, key components of effective programs, and strategies for promoting continuous learning and professional development in medication safety [13].

10.1 Importance of education and training

Education and training in medication safety are essential for several reasons:

- Enhancing knowledge: healthcare professionals need a solid foundation of knowledge regarding medication safety principles, best practices, and relevant regulations and guidelines.

- Improving skills: training programs can help develop and refine skills such as medication calculation, compounding, administration, and error prevention techniques.

- Promoting awareness: education raises awareness about the potential risks associated with medication administration in neonatal care, fostering a culture of vigilance and accountability.
- Ensuring competency: competency-based education and training programs ensure that healthcare professionals possess the necessary skills and knowledge to provide safe medication practices.

10.2 Key components of education and training programs

Effective education and training programs in medication safety should incorporate the following components:

- Curriculum development: developing a comprehensive curriculum that covers essential topics such as medication safety principles, medication administration techniques, error prevention strategies, and high-risk medications.
- Evidence-based content: ensuring that the education and training materials are based on the latest research, guidelines, and best practices in medication safety.
- Practical training: providing hands-on training opportunities, simulation exercises, and case studies that allow healthcare professionals to apply their knowledge in realistic scenarios.
- Interprofessional collaboration: promoting collaboration and communication among healthcare professionals from different disciplines involved in medication administration, including pharmacists, nurses, and physicians.
- Ongoing assessment and evaluation: implementing assessments and evaluations to measure the effectiveness of the education and training programs and identify areas for improvement.

10.3 Strategies for continuous learning and professional development

Continuous learning and professional development are essential to ensure that healthcare professionals stay updated with the latest advancements and best practices in medication safety. Strategies to promote continuous learning include:

- Continuing education programs: offering opportunities for healthcare professionals to attend workshops, conferences, webinars, and seminars focused on medication safety.
- Access to resources: providing access to online databases, journals, guidelines, and educational materials related to medication safety.
- Peer learning and mentoring: encouraging healthcare professionals to engage in peer discussions, case reviews, and mentorship programs to share experiences and learn from one another.
- Quality improvement initiatives: participating in quality improvement projects and initiatives focused on medication safety, such as medication error reduction programs and medication safety committees.

- Incorporating technology: leveraging technology platforms, such as e-learning modules and mobile applications, to facilitate convenient and accessible learning opportunities.

10.4 Integration into practice

Education and training in medication safety should not only be limited to theoretical knowledge but also emphasize its practical application in clinical settings. Strategies for integrating education and training into practice include:

- Preceptorship and mentorship programs: pairing novice healthcare professionals with experienced mentors who can provide guidance and support in medication safety practices.
- Standard operating procedures: developing standardized protocols and guidelines for medication administration, including error prevention strategies and safety measures.
- Regular competency assessments: conducting periodic competency assessments to ensure healthcare professionals maintain the necessary skills and knowledge in medication safety.
- Feedback and performance reviews: providing regular feedback and performance reviews to identify areas for improvement and recognize excellence in medication safety practices.

By investing in comprehensive education and training programs, healthcare organizations can empower their professionals to provide safe and effective medication practices in neonatal care. Continuous learning, professional development, and a commitment to ongoing improvement are essential for ensuring optimal medication safety and enhancing patient outcomes in this vulnerable population [3, 7, 13].

11. Conclusion

In neonatal care, medication safety is a vital shield against errors and adverse events. This chapter has explored the unique challenges and essential strategies in this field.

Neonates, particularly premature infants, demand a precise and safety-oriented approach to medication. Understanding nuances from prescribing to administration, including accurate dosing and personalized regimens, is paramount.

Throughout our exploration, we have stressed proper medication storage, labeling, and adherence to expiration dates. We've also covered critical topics like medication reconciliation, route-specific safety, dosage calculations, and technology use.

For high-risk medications, we have discussed vigilant monitoring, dose adjustments, and precise administration techniques. Embracing technology, like barcode scanning and smart infusion pumps, bolsters safety.

We've also emphasized the importance of reporting and learning from medication errors, fostering a culture of improvement. Education, ongoing training, and competency assessment are vital.

In closing, our journey equips us with a solid foundation for safer medication use and a commitment to quality neonatal care through collaboration and vigilance.

Author details

Hossam A. Elgnainy
Clinical Pharmacist at Cairo University Specialized Pediatric Hospital, Egypt

*Address all correspondence to: helgnainy@gmail.com

References

[1] Krzyzaniak N, Bajorek B. Medication safety in neonatal care: A review of medication errors among neonates. Therapeutic Advances in Drug Safety. 2016;**7**(3):102-119

[2] Dabliz R, Levine S. Medication safety in neonates. American Journal of Perinatology. 2012;**29**(01):49-56

[3] Santesteban E, Arenas S, Campino A. Medication errors in neonatal care: A systematic review of types of errors and effectiveness of preventive strategies. Journal of Neonatal Nursing. 2015;**21**(5):200-208

[4] Holmes AP. NICU Primer for pharmacists. ASHP; 2015. Available from: https://store.ashp.org/Default.aspx?TabID=251&productId=324860061. eBook E4771; eISBN: 978-1-58528-477-1

[5] Greenberg RG, Smith PB, Bose C, Clark RH, Cotten CM, DeRienzo C. National survey of neonatal intensive care unit medication safety practices. American Journal of Perinatology. 2018;**35**(14):1419-1422

[6] Kuitunen S. Medication safety in intravenous drug administration: Error causes and systemic defenses in hospital setting. Terveyden tutkimuksen tutkijakoulun väitöskirjasarja (59/2022). 2022. Available from: https://helda.helsinki.fi/items/5441c513-bff7-4d79-b448-98954e2064a7. ISBN 978-951-51-8563-1 (online)

[7] Chedoe I, Molendijk H, Hospes W, Van den Heuvel ER, Taxis K. The effect of a multifaceted educational intervention on medication preparation and administration errors in neonatal intensive care. Archives of Disease in Childhood-Fetal and Neonatal Edition. 2012;**97**(6):F449-F455

[8] Kunac DL, Reith DM. Identification of priorities for medication safety in neonatal intensive care. Drug Safety. 2005;**28**:251-261

[9] Melton KR, Timmons K, Walsh KE, Meinzen-Derr JK, Kirkendall E. Smart pumps improve medication safety but increase alert burden in neonatal care. BMC Medical Informatics and Decision Making. 2019;**19**(1):1-1

[10] Stokowski LA. Using technology to improve medication safety in the newborn intensive care unit. Advances in Neonatal Care. 2001;**1**(2):70-83

[11] Whalen K, Lynch E, Moawad I, John T, Lozowski D, Cummings BM. Transition to a new electronic health record and pediatric medication safety: Lessons learned in pediatrics within a large academic health system. Journal of the American Medical Informatics Association. 2018;**25**(7):848-854

[12] Cronje L. Intravenous Medication Safety Practices of Registered Nurses in Neonatal and Paediatric Critical Care Areas [doctoral dissertation]. Stellenbosch: Stellenbosch University; 2012

[13] Marufu TC, Bower R, Hendron E, Manning JC. Nursing interventions to reduce medication errors in paediatrics and neonates: Systematic review and meta-analysis. Journal of Pediatric Nursing. 2022;**62**:e139-e147

[14] Miller LE, DeRienzo C, Smith PB, Bose C, Clark RH, Cotten CM, et al. Association between neonatal intensive care unit medication safety practices, adverse events, and death. Journal of Perinatology. 2021;**41**(7):1739-1744

Chapter 10

Risks Versus Benefits of Using Aspirin, Magnesium Sulfate, Corticosteroids, and Progesterone during Pregnancy

Enrique Valdés Rubio and Osvaldo Flores Belkerbach

Abstract

This chapter will discuss various prophylactic and therapeutic strategies based on a review of the literature that is based on the best evidence. In this way, we will know the effect of aspirin as a prophylactic measure in the prevention of severe preeclampsia. Then, we treat the impact of magnesium sulfate to significantly reduce intracranial hemorrhage and cerebral palsy. Following this, we examine the impact of corticosteroids in premature pregnancies in different clinical scenarios, demonstrating their efficacy in improving neonatal prognosis. Finally, we will see the effect of progesterone in reducing premature labor. The use of these strategies has allowed for an improvement in perinatal morbidity and mortality due to the intrinsic beneficial effects of these drugs, as well as a decrease in prematurity (aspirin and progesterone).

Keywords: prevention in pregnancy, corticosteroids, progesterone, aspirin, magnesium sulfate

1. Introduction

Recently, several prophylactic strategies for preventing poor perinatal outcomes have been studied. Thus, in this chapter we will share the four biomedical interventions that have proven to be safe and effective for improving neonatal prognosis, despite their contradictory evidence, and except for when corticosteroids are indicated. Next, we will review the effect of corticosteroids, progesterone, aspirin and magnesium sulfate by reviewing the literature based on the available evidence.

2. Aspirin: Acetylsalicylic acid

2.1 History

Aspirin is one of the oldest medications still in use in the modern world. The first records of "salix", a component of aspirin derived from willow bark, were found in papyri used by Egyptian physicians in 1534 BC [1]. Hippocrates also recommended herbal tea made from white willow leaves for pain and fever. Hundreds of years later, in 1829, Pierre Leroux obtained salicin crystals by boiling white willow bark powder. Later, in 1842, Raffaele Piria synthesized salicylic acid for the first time, however, it had many adverse effects. In 1953, Gerhardt was the first to isolate acetylsalicylic acid as we know it today [2].

In 1971, Vane, Samuelson, and Bergstrom were awarded the Nobel Prize for elucidating aspirin's mechanism of action and they initiated the clinical research on its antiplatelet effects [1]. This last effect has made aspirin one of the most prescribed medications in the world and it is taken by more than 50 million people to prevent cardiovascular disease.

In the field of prenatal care, aspirin appeared for the first time in 1978 in a case reported by Goodlin et al. They describe a patient with a history of two premature births due to hypertensive crises and thrombocytopenia (currently HELLP syndrome) who was undergoing her third pregnancy with similar characteristics. At 15 weeks, she already presented thrombocytopenia, so after a course of heparin with no favorable results, aspirin was started given its antiplatelet effect. The patient had a remission of her plateletopenia and reached 34 weeks of gestation resulting in a live newborn weighing 1410 grams [3]. Shortly thereafter, in 1978, in the wake of this case report, Crandon et al. published a retrospective study that demonstrated that aspirin could have a role in the prevention of preeclampsia [4]. In the following years, multiple studies were published on the protective role of aspirin in hypertensive disorders of pregnancy.

2.2 Preeclampsia

Preeclampsia is a multifactorial systemic disorder, which occurs syndromatically. It is characterized by high blood pressure associated with proteinuria and/or the dysfunction of an organ or system. It affects between 3 to 5% of all pregnancies, representing one of the main causes of maternal morbidity and mortality, especially when it begins early on in pregnancy [5, 6]. Of all premature births, one-sixth are due to preeclampsia; and out of all preeclampsias, a third must be interrupted before term with all the morbidity and mortality associated with newborn prematurity [6]. This is the reason why it is important to have predictive methods for preeclampsia and, concomitantly, to have a prevention strategy, which is where the role of aspirin arises.

2.3 Pathophysiology of preeclampsia and mechanism of action of aspirin

PE is characterized by a systemic proinflammatory state in which cytokines, free radicals, oxidized lipids, oxygen reactive species, and sFlt-1 are released into circulation, among other molecules that cause the clinical characteristics observed in PE. This endothelial dysfunction causes an increase in the peroxidation of endothelial lipids and these, in turn, activate the cyclooxygenase (COX) enzyme and inhibit prostacyclin synthase, enzymes that regulate the production of prostaglandins that play a leading role in the pathophysiology of PE [7]. Prostaglandins are fat-soluble molecules that participate in multiple biological processes, both physiological and pathological. They are synthesized from arachidonic acid (AA) which is present in practically all cells by means of the COX enzyme. This enzyme converts AA into prostaglandin H_2 which is metabolized into several other types of prostaglandins depending on the cell type in which the reaction occurs and the type of enzyme that acts upon it. Prostacyclin synthase, present mainly in endothelial cells, transforms AA into prostacyclins (prostaglandin I2) which have a vasodilatory effect and inhibit platelet aggregation and adhesion. On the other hand, thromboxane synthase produces thromboxane from AA. It is found mainly in platelets and causes a vasoconstrictor effect, contrary to prostacyclins [8]. Aspirin induces the acetylation of a serine in the COX enzyme, binding irreversibly to its catalytic site. This prevents the binding of AA which causes an inhibition of its action. Although aspirin irreversibly blocks the action of COX in its production of endothelial prostacyclin as platelet thromboxane, endothelial cells quickly activate gene mechanisms that allow new COX to be produced, which allows normal levels of prostacyclins to be maintained. On the other hand, platelets that do not have a nucleus cannot activate genetic mechanisms that generate new COX molecules for the production of thromboxane. This imbalance causes disequilibrium in the thromboxane/prostacyclin balance in favor of the latter, which would generate a protective effect by reducing the inflammation previously described in the pathophysiology of PE [7, 9]. These findings have been corroborated in studies that show that patients with PE have high levels of thromboxane and low levels of prostacyclins [10]. This imbalance can already be seen during the first trimester of pregnancy, and studies show that when aspirin is administered, this imbalance is reversed after 2 weeks, favoring vasodilation in the systemic circulation, specifically in the remodeling of the spiral arteries. In addition, there is a decrease in antiangiogenic factors such as sFlt-1 and an increase in circulating levels of PlGF [2].

In summary, the effect of aspirin in the prevention of preeclampsia is due to an improvement in the placentation process, the inhibition of platelet aggregation, and its antithrombotic effect which leads to lower levels of placental infarction, its anti-inflammatory effects, and endothelial stabilization [6].

2.4 Aspirin and prevention of preeclampsia

As already mentioned, since the late 1970s, multiple studies have been published regarding the prevention of preeclampsia with the use of aspirin, however, the results have varied, and even contradictory. This variation in results is likely due to the heterogeneity in the methodology of the studies in addition to the multifactorial etiopathogenesis of preeclampsia. This heterogeneity includes:

- Patient selection: There are several ways to stratify the risk of developing preeclampsia and therefore prescribe the use of aspirin to a particular patient. Different studies and international societies apply very diverse criteria to classify patients who are at risk. For example, some are founded on assigning a score based on major risk factors or a sum of lesser risk factors [11–13]. Other guidelines have assigned value to an altered uterine artery Doppler in the first trimester, without considering other risk factors [14]. In other latitudes, patients are stratified based on an algorithm that assigns a specific risk according to the presence or absence of several environmental and biophysical variables [15].

- Aspirin dose: another possible cause of the variation of the results is that the only thing that all the studies coincide on is to administrate of low doses of aspirin.

However, these low doses have been studied with 50 mg, 60 mg, 75 mg, 81, 100 mg, or 150 mg [15–19].

- Gestational age at the time of indicating or stopping aspirin: another point of controversy is when the indication of aspirin starts. Several authors indicated the use of aspirin anytime a risk factor for preeclampsia was observed, regardless of gestational age. Others, on the other hand, started aspirin in the first trimester, and others before 16 or 20 weeks [15, 18, 20, 21]. In the 2010s, important meta-analyses were published regarding the use of aspirin in PE prevention, one of them showed that a greater decrease in the appearance of preeclampsia is achieved when aspirin is started before 16 weeks of gestation [22]. The same group later went on to demonstrate through another meta-analysis that starting aspirin before 16 weeks only achieves the desired effect in preventing the preeclampsia that appears before term (37 weeks) and does not influence the prevention of pre-eclampsia that begins after this gestational age [23]. Finally, a more recent meta-analysis by the same group reported that the dose of aspirin does influence the results, demonstrating greater benefits in studies that used higher doses of aspirin (150 mg) [24]. In 2017, as a result of the publications of these meta-analyses, a large randomized controlled trial was published, which showed that in patients at a high risk of preeclampsia, the use of aspirin indicated before 16 weeks of pregnancy, at a dose of 150 mg per night (circadian effect), decreased the rate of preterm preeclampsia by 62% (OR 0.38; 95% CI, 0.20–0.74; p = .004) [15].

Despite the evidence shown in the prior paragraph, the different large obstetrics and gynecology societies still have not agreed on the criteria regarding when aspirin should be initiated, what the recommended dose is, and when its use should be stopped, as shown in **Table 1**.

Other beneficial effects of aspirin have been studied and have demonstrated a decrease in poor obstetric outcomes such as the restriction of intrauterine growth, in-utero fetal death, and admission to neonatal intensive care units. However, the studies have more biases and less statistical power, so better quality studies are required in order to be able to provide a recommendation [6].

Guide	Start of aspirin use	Dose	Cessation of use
ACOG	12–28 weeks. Ideally before 16 weeks	81 mg	Until childbirth
RCOG	12 weeks	150 mg or 2 tablets of 81 mg (acceptable)	Until childbirth
WHO	<20 weeks	75 mg	Unspecified
FIGO	11–14 + 6 weeks	150 mg	Up to 36 weeks, or when preeclampsia is diagnosed
NICE	12 weeks	75 mg at moderate risk and 150 mg at high risk	Until childbirth

ACOG: American College of Obstetricians and Gynecologist, RCOG: Royal College of Obstetricians and Gynecologist; WHO: World Health Organization; FIGO: International Federation of Gynecology and Obstetrics; and NICE: National Institute of Health Organization. Adapted from Horgan et al. [25].

Table 1.
Recommendations from different scientific societies regarding the use of aspirin.

3. Magnesium sulfate

Magnesium Sulfate in the obstetric field is relevant due to its tocolytic effect (prevention of premature birth), prophylaxis, and treatment of eclampsia in severe hypertensive conditions (effect on maternal morbidity) as well as its role in reducing cerebral palsy in premature newborns. This section will focus on this last role.

3.1 Cerebral paralysis

It is a spectrum of non-progressive movement and posture disorders that have multiple causes, clinical types, and degrees of severity. It is also associated with intellectual disability, autism, epilepsy, and visual impairment [26]. It has an approximate incidence between 2 and 2.5/1000 births, with a relationship that is inversely proportional to the gestational age at birth, both in its incidence and in its degree of severity. Some series reported that a quarter of newborns with cerebral palsy were born before 34 weeks and a third of babies with cerebral palsy born before 26 weeks cannot walk [26–28]. Neonatal encephalopathy secondary to injury or acute peripartum hypoxia is often attributed as the cause of cerebral palsy; however, only 13% of term newborns diagnosed with neonatal encephalopathy subsequently developed cerebral palsy [29]. In its pathophysiology, cerebral palsy is observed in the context of a diffuse white matter lesion or cystic periventricular leukomalacia, or both. It may also be seen as intraventricular hemorrhage. Lesions have been described in the corticospinal tract, as well as in the posterior thalamic radiations connecting the thalamus with the occipital and posterior parietal cortex. Neuronal loss has also been described in the subplate, basal ganglia, and cerebellum [30].

Risk factors associated with cerebral palsy are, as already mentioned, premature birth, coexisting congenital anomalies, intrauterine infections, abnormal fetal inflammatory response, thrombophilia, intrauterine growth restriction, multiple pregnancies, circular nuchal cord tension during childbirth, prolonged shoulder dystocia, placental pathology, congenital errors of metabolism, genetic factors that cause intrinsic brain damage or increased susceptibility to brain injury, and finally a greater association with the male sex [26].

3.2 Magnesium sulfate as cerebral palsy prophylaxis

Magnesium Sulfate has been used for several decades in the prevention and treatment of eclampsia. In the early 1990s, a retrospective observational study described that women who received magnesium sulfate, in the context of a hypertensive syndrome of pregnancy, demonstrated a decrease in the incidence of cerebral palsy in premature babies, particularly those patients who did not have preeclampsia [31]. Based on these findings, the role of magnesium sulfate in the prophylaxis of cerebral palsy began to be actively studied. Thus, in the 2000s, 5 large studies appeared that tried to demonstrate the relationship in the decrease of cerebral palsy with magnesium sulfate when it was administered in the context of premature birth [32–36]. In most of them, the primary results that tried to demonstrate that magnesium sulfate decreased cerebral palsy were not met. However, a meta-analysis that included these 5 large trials demonstrated that there were no differences in terms of pediatric mortality between exposed and unexposed children (RR 1.04, 95% CI, 0.82–1.17). However, evidence of a relative decrease in cerebral palsy of 32% was observed (RR 0.68, 95% CI, 0.54–0.87). Sixty-three had to be treated to prevent one case of cerebral palsy (95% CI, 39–172) [37]. In addition, there was evidence of a significant decrease in gross motor dysfunction (RR 0.61, 95% CI, 0.44–0.85).

Subsequent follow-up studies in school-aged children did not demonstrate harmful effects in children exposed to magnesium sulfate, which is why it is currently considered a safe therapy [35, 38]. A more recent Cochrane review that evaluated different measures for preventing cerebral palsy reported that the use of magnesium sulfate has high-quality evidence in fetal neuroprotection, unlike other prophylactic measures [39].

Regarding its physiological mechanism of action, magnesium is an important mediator in cellular apoptosis pathways that occur during inflammatory processes. It competitively reduces calcium entry into the cell, blocks glutamate and other excitatory neurotransmitters, and modulates the actions of proinflammatory cytokines and oxygen free radicals. Furthermore, magnesium is considered a vasoactive agent, with hemodynamic benefits in the fetus and newborn which include the stabilization of blood pressure and cerebral arterial perfusion [40].

3.3 Practical considerations regarding magnesium sulfate

There are no clear definitions regarding the time when magnesium sulfate should be administrated given the heterogeneity of the different studies; however, most international guidelines agree on administering it in the face of imminent delivery before 30–32 weeks of gestation. The doses also usually vary, nevertheless, the most commonly used corresponds to a loading dose of 4 grams to be administered in 30 minutes followed by a continuous infusion of 1 gram/hour administered for 24 hours or until the child is born. As an exception, its use can be extended in cases of prophylaxis for postpartum eclampsia. It is recommended to monitor the mother with clinical parameters due to the risk of poisoning, through the serial assessment of diuresis, tendon reflexes, respiratory rate, and state of consciousness. Regarding its concomitant use with other tocolytics, recommendations differ [41].

4. Corticosteroids

The beneficial effect of corticosteroids in animals has been recognized for more than 50 years. Liggins was the first to conduct experiments on sheep, concluding that premature lambs exposed to corticosteroids had a better survival prognosis than those that had not received them. In 1972, this same author, together with Howie, published the first randomized controlled study of the effect of corticosteroids in humans concluding that corticosteroids not only reduced the risk of respiratory distress syndrome (RDS) (from 25.8 to 9%) but also significantly reduced neonatal mortality (15 to 3.2%) [42]. Finally, it is interesting to note that a meta-analysis that included more than 1400 pregnant women with premature rupture of membranes (PROM) who received a single dose of corticosteroids showed that RDS decreased significantly (RR 0.56, 95% CI 46–70), HIV (RR 0.47, 98% CI 0.31–0.70 CI) and EN (RR 0.21, 95% CI 0.05–0.82) [43]. The evidence with the most statistical power and with a high degree of recommendation is a Cochrane systematic review that included 30 studies that encompassed 7774 pregnant women and 8158 neonates whose mothers had mostly received a course of corticosteroids (betamethasone, dexamethasone, or hydrocortisone) except 9 trials in which a second course was administered 7 days apart compared with a placebo or no treatment. This regimen was indicated for women with a single or multiple pregnancy, before premature birth occurred (elective or after spontaneous labor), regardless of another comorbidity. This meta-analysis highlights that prenatal corticosteroid treatment (compared with a placebo or no treatment) is associated with a decrease in the most serious adverse outcomes related to prematurity which include: perinatal death, neonatal death, RDS, wet lung, necrotizing enterocolitis, periventricular leukomalacia and less need for mechanical ventilation (less use of surfactant and neonatal infections in the first 48 hours) [42–44].

4.1 Physiological effect of antenatal corticosteroids

The use of corticosteroids in premature pregnancies decreases mortality and respiratory distress syndrome. The physiological mechanism of how corticosteroid therapy would act would be through the stimulation of surfactant production by type 2 pneumocytes, the maturing of connective tissue, and the stimulation the synthesis of elastin.

Betamethasone (two doses of 12 mg intramuscularly every 24 hours) and dexamethasone (four doses of 6 mg every 12 hours) are the corticosteroids prescribed for the prenatal period due to a series of advantages. The most noteworthy are that these corticosteroids pass through the placenta without losing effectiveness and this lasts even after delivery since newborns respond better to the effect of postnatal surfactant and furthermore, the effect on neonatal plasma is short, no more than 40 hours after delivery.

Betamethasone and dexamethasone are the most widely studied corticosteroids and, in general, have been preferred as prenatal treatment to decrease neonatal death and to accelerate the maturing of other fetal organs (not only the fetal lung) since a decrease in HIV, periventricular leukomalacia and necrotizing enterocolitis became evident. Both pass through the placenta in their active form and have almost identical biological activity.

4.2 Impact of corticosteroids on perinatal outcome

The accumulated evidence advises the use of a course of corticosteroids in pregnant women who have a threat of premature birth between 24/0 weeks and 33/6 weeks of pregnancy and who have a real risk of delivering within 7 days [43, 44].

Besides, the use of corticosteroids in patients with premature rupture of membranes (RPM) between the weeks already indicated has proven its indication, not only in improving respiratory morbidity. If not, mortality, intraventricular hemorrhage, and necrotizing enterocolitis have also decreased [45–47].

In relation to the probable risk that corticosteroids have in facilitating infectious processes, it has been published that their use in pregnant women with PROM does not increase infection in the mother-child binomial, and their indication can even be considered from week 230/7 and that they are giving birth within 7 days [43, 48]. .Repetitive use or a rescue course of corticosteroids with preterm PROM is controversial, as there is not enough evidence to make a recommendation for or against it.

The studies that support the use of corticosteroids in pregnancy are contradictory; in fact, Cochrane concludes that more studies are needed to suggest their indication. Despite the above, a retrospective study was recently published that indicated that prenatal corticosteroids in twin pregnancies within 7 days before delivery were associated with a significant reduction in premature neonatal pathology (neonatal mortality, neurological injury, and respiratory distress) [43, 44, 49, 50].

In relation to imminent late preterm birth, recent data also suggest that betamethasone may be beneficial in pregnant women at high risk of late preterm birth, between 34 0/7 weeks and 36 6/7 weeks of gestation who have not received a prior course of prenatal. To answer this hypothesis, a study led by The Maternal-Fetal Medicine Units Network Antenatal Late Preterm Steroids Trial was carried out. This study was a randomized, double-blind, placebo-controlled clinical trial designed to evaluate the use of prenatal betamethasone in pregnant women at a high risk of delivery in the late preterm period. Women were identified as being high risk if they were in preterm labor, had preterm PROM, or had a planned delivery in the late preterm period, with the indication at the discretion of the obstetrician-gynecologist or other health care provider. Tocolysis was not used as part of this trial and delivery was not delayed due to obstetric or medical indications. The study found that betamethasone administration led to a significant decrease in the primary outcome, which was the need for respiratory support. A greater decrease was demonstrated for serious respiratory complications, from 12.1% in the placebo group to 8.1% in the betamethasone group (RR, 0.67; 95% CI, 0.53–0.84; $P < 0.001$). There were also significant decreases in rates of transient tachypnea in newborns; bronchopulmonary dysplasia; a combination of respiratory distress syndrome (RDS), transient tachypnea in the newborn and RDS; and the need for postnatal surfactant. Infants exposed to betamethasone were less likely to require immediate postnatal resuscitation. There was no increase in proven neonatal sepsis, chorioamnionitis, or endometritis with betamethasone in the late preterm period. Hypoglycemia was more common in betamethasone-exposed infants 24.0% versus 14.9% (RR, 1.61; 95% CI, 1.38–1.88); however, no adverse events related to hypoglycemia were reported, and neither an increase in the length of hospital stay. The rates of hypoglycemia found in the trial are similar to those reported in the general population of late preterm infants [51–53]. Currently, there is greater evidence supporting the use of corticosteroids in late preterm infants, particularly in those women who had not received a prior course.

Finally, ACOG recommended that elective cesarean sections should be performed at 39 weeks to reduce potential risks associated with prematurity in newborns at 38 weeks. Therefore, we hypothesize that the 38-week-old fetus needs labor to release corticosteroids and other mediators that would reduce neonatal complications associated with prematurity. In this way, the authors of this chapter carried out a randomized case-control study in which some patients received a course of corticosteroids at 37 + 5 and 37 + 6 and were operated on at 38 weeks, and the controls at 39 weeks who did not receive this indication. The results of this study are encouraging, because they show that in selected cases and exceptionally, the administration of corticosteroids at 38 weeks prior to an elective cesarean section does not have worse results than an elective cesarean section at 39 weeks (RDS 0% vs. 1.1%, $p = 1.0$, transient tachypnea 0% vs. 0% and admission to neonatal intensive care unit 8.8% vs. 6.3%, $p = 0.7$) [54].

Finally, there are still no methodologically well-done studies in the literature to advise that cycles less than or equal to two doses present any risk of alteration of neurobehavioral development. Therefore, the 2000 NICHD consensus panel concluded that studies on the possible benefits and risks of repeated courses of prenatal corticosteroids are limited due to their designs and "methodological inconsistencies." It also noted that while there is a suggestion of a possible benefit of repeated courses (especially in the decrease and severity of respiratory distress), there is also data in animals and humans suggesting deleterious effects on the fetus with regards to myelination of the brain, lungs, growth, and function of the hypothalamic-pituitary-adrenal axis. Follow-up of children at 2 years of age who were exposed to repeated courses of prenatal corticosteroids showed no significant differences in physical or neurocognitive measurements in two studies [55, 56], and the same result was found in younger children in a third study. Although not statistically significant, the relative risk of cerebral palsy in infants exposed to a series of prenatal corticosteroids (RR, 5.7; 95% confidence interval, 0.7–46.7; P = 0.12) as observed in one study is a cause for concern and warrants further study. Maternal effects include a greater risk of infection and suppression of the hypothalamic-pituitary-adrenal axis [57]. Regularly scheduled repeat cycles or serial cycles (more than two) are currently not recommended [58].

5. Progesterone

Preterm birth is the most frequent complication in Maternal-Fetal Medicine with an incidence ranging from 6.5% to 12.5% depending on the different regions of the world and it is the main cause of morbidity and mortality in the neonate. Research on this condition is a priority for the World Health Organization (WHO) and it is considered key for decreasing prenatal deaths by the United Nations [59].

Despite being controversial, one of the strategies that has proven its effectiveness is progesterone.

This hormone, in both its presentations as micronized natural progesterone and 17 alpha hydroxyprogesterone caproate (c17-OHP), has as a possible mechanism of action, an anti-inflammatory effect. It may also maintain the myometrium quiescent, decrease the degradation of the cervical stroma, decrease the contractile frequency of the uterus, attenuate the decidual hemorrhage/inflammation response, and inhibit connexin-43. However, it should be kept in mind that although both presentations are types of progesterone, current evidence concludes that only micronized natural progesterone decreases the contractility of the myometrium and prevents cervical modifications whereas c17-OHP would not do so since it would act by different pathophysiological mechanisms [59].

5.1 Impact of progesterone in pregnant women with a prior history of premature birth

Regarding c17-OHP, in pregnant women with a previous history of preterm birth and singleton pregnancy, both the first clinical trials [30] and a subsequent meta-analysis reported a significant decrease in delivery <37 weeks and in perinatal morbidity after the prophylactic administration of c17-OHP (intramuscular [IM] at a dose of 250 mg every 7 days). The greatest effectiveness was observed when its administration was started before 21 weeks of gestation (usually from 16 to 20 weeks to week 36). Notwithstanding, the risk of gestational diabetes tripled in the pregnant women who were studied [31].

The study that refuted the efficacy and safety of the latter was the one published in 2020 (PROLONG [32], a randomized, multicenter, placebo-controlled trial that evaluates the safety and efficacy of c17-OHP injections in 1707 pregnant women with a singleton pregnancy and a history of prior preterm delivery. This study did not demonstrate that c17-OHP decreases delivery <35 weeks (11.0 vs. 11.5%; RR 0.95; 95% CI: 0.71–1.26), nor neonatal morbidity (5.6 vs. 5.0%; RR 1.12; 95% CI: 0.68–1.61), nor fetal/early infant death (1.7 vs. 1.9%; RR 0.87; 95% CI: 0.40–1.81). Maternal outcomes were also similar between the 2 groups.

In twin pregnancies, two randomized (double-blind, placebo-controlled) studies revealed that c17-OHP did not reduce the risk of preterm birth nor improve fetal or neonatal outcomes [33, 34].

On the other hand, natural micronized progesterone would not reduce the risk of birth <34, <37 weeks nor improve neonatal morbidity and mortality in pregnant women with a history of prior preterm birth and normal cervical length [35, 36]. Supporting this conclusion, the PROGRESS study [37] (randomizing 787 pregnant women with a single or twin pregnancy and a history of prior preterm birth) evaluated the effectiveness of a progesterone pessary (equivalent to 100 mg of vaginal micronized progesterone) vs. a placebo and did not observe a decrease in labor <37 weeks (adjusted RR 0.97; 95% CI: 0.81–1.17), nor in the risk of neonatal respiratory distress (adjusted RR 0.98; 95% CI: 0.82–1.17) or other neonatal or maternal outcomes related to preterm birth (adjusted RR 1.35; 95% CI: 0.85–2.15).

Finally, in the OPPTIMUM study [35] no differences were observed when the efficacy of progesterone was evaluated in pregnant women at a high risk of preterm birth (odds ratio [OR] 0.86 [95% CI: 0.61–1.22]). Therefore, administration of c17-OHP or vaginal micronized natural progesterone to prevent preterm birth is not recommended solely because of the history of previous preterm birth.

5.2 Impact of progesterone in singleton pregnancies and short cervix

c17-OHP does not decrease the risk of preterm birth in pregnancies with a short cervix (cervical length ≤ 25 mm) [60]. Regarding natural micronized vaginal progesterone, in pregnant women with a short cervix, with or without a history of preterm birth, it has been reported that progesterone is effective in decreasing preterm birth <34 weeks [35, 38] (RR 0.60; 95% CI: 0.44–0.82) neonatal complications (neonatal respiratory distress (RR 0.47; 95% CI: 0.27–0.81) and neonatal morbidity and mortality (RR 0.59; 95% CI: 0 .38–0.91) with the number of pregnant women that need to be treated being 10 (95% CI: 7–28), 18 (95% CI: 13–51) and 18 (95% CI: 12–81) respectively [61]. The benefit would not depend on the maternal age, BMI, race, or ethnicity.

However, the OPPTIMUM [60] study published later contradicts the results of previous meta-analyses. In said study, the pregnant women who were selected had a high risk of preterm birth (history of preterm birth <34 weeks and/or cervix <25 mm). They were randomized to receive 200 mg daily of vaginal progesterone vs. placebo with administration starting at weeks 22–24 through week 34. The study did not observe a decrease in preterm birth nor any improvement in perinatal outcomes in the vaginal progesterone group. Subsequently, another meta-analysis [62] (5 studies, 974 pregnant women) confirmed the results of the previous meta-analyses regarding the benefit of progesterone in reducing labor <34 weeks (RR 0.72; 95% CI: 0.55–0.95). No differences were observed regarding the neurodevelopment of those born after 2 years of follow-up. Therefore, the administration of natural micronized progesterone (200 mg/24 h vaginally) is recommended in asymptomatic pregnant women with singleton pregnancies and a short cervix (≤ 25 mm) to prevent preterm birth, regardless of whether they have a history of previous preterm birth or not.

5.3 Impact of progesterone in twin pregnancies

If the current evidence is taken into account, progesterone has not been shown to decrease preterm birth in twin pregnancies [63]. This conclusion is supported by a Cochrane review [64] that analyzed the effectiveness of progesterone (both vaginal and IM) as prophylaxis in twin pregnancies (16 randomized studies with placebo, 4548 pregnant women). A higher percentage of delivery <34 weeks was observed in the group treated with c17-OHP than in the placebo group (RR 1.54; 95% CI: 1.06–2.26). With regards to vaginal progesterone, no significant differences were observed in the risk of preterm birth (RR 0.90; 95% CI: 0.66–1.23), nor in neonatal morbidity-mortality. Finally, in pregnant women with twin pregnancies and a short cervix, Romero et al. [58], in a meta-analysis with six randomized clinical trials that included pregnant women with twin pregnancies and cervical length < 25 mm, observed that vaginal progesterone decreased labor <33 weeks (31.4% vs. 43.1%; RR 0 .69; 95% CI: 0.51–0.93) and neonatal morbidity and mortality, without finding differences in the neurodevelopment of these children at 4–5 years of follow-up. Currently, the data from this study is being analyzed once again and these results are pending. For now, there is not enough evidence to recommend the use of vaginal micronized progesterone in twin pregnancies.

6. Conclusions

The use of the interventions described in this chapter has been shown to decrease perinatal morbidity and mortality. Their application is recommended in all clinical settings due to their easy applicability, and excellent cost-effectiveness due to the low cost of these pharmacological therapies compared to the great expense generated by caring for a premature newborn, both in the short and long term.

With regards to the use of aspirin, there is a consensus that its use started before 16 weeks, in a high-risk population, with doses greater than 100 mg, significantly reduces the risk of preeclampsia, and to a lesser extent the risk of restriction of fetal growth.

Regarding the use of magnesium sulfate, although the evidence is more limited, its use is currently suggested to reduce the risk of cerebral palsy, when there is an imminent risk of premature birth before 32 weeks. After this gestational age, its use does not have significant benefits.

Regarding corticosteroids, a single course of corticosteroids has immediate and substantial benefits in immature fetuses between 24 and 33 + 6 days in pregnant women who present a high risk of giving birth within 7 days, both in the premature rupture of membranes as well as in twin pregnancies. A second course or a rescue dose in pregnancies less than 34 weeks, at risk of delivering within 7 days, whose first course was indicated 7 to 14 days after receiving the first dose, has also been seen to be beneficial. The indication of a second dose in pregnant women with PROM, as well as its use in pregnancies between 34 + 0–36 + 6 weeks, still has limited evidence. Finally, there is evidence in the literature that supports the indication of a course of corticosteroids in women undergoing an elective cesarean section at 38 weeks in exceptional situations.

Finally, the use of vaginal progesterone has been shown to reduce the incidence of premature birth in those women who have a singleton pregnancy, with a history of premature birth and a short cervix. The use of progesterone in twin pregnancies does not have enough evidence to make a recommendation.

Conflict of interest

The authors declare no conflict of interest.

Author details

Enrique Valdés Rubio[1,2*] and Osvaldo Flores Belkerbach[1]

1 Hospital Clínico Universidad de Chile, Santiago, Chile

2 Universidad Andrés Bello, Chile

*Address all correspondence to: e.valdes.r.63@gmail.com

References

[1] Navaratnam K, Alfirevic A, Alfirevic Z. Low dose aspirin and pregnancy: How important is aspirin resistance? BJOG. 2016;**123**:1481-1487

[2] Atallah A, Lecarpentier E, Goffinet F, et al. Aspirin for prevention of preeclampsia. Drugs. 2017;**77**:1819

[3] Goodlin RC, Haesslein HO, Fleming J. Aspirin for the treatment of recurrent toxaemia. Lancet. 1978;**2**:51

[4] Crandon AJ, Isherwood DM. Effect of aspirin on incidence of pre-eclampsia. Lancet. 1979;**1**:1356

[5] Abalos E, Cuesta C, Grosso AL, et al. Global and regional estimates of preeclampsia and eclampsia: A systematic review. European Journal of Obstetrics, Gynecology, and Reproductive Biology. 2013;**170**:1-7

[6] Rolnik DL, Nicolaides KH, Poon LC. Prevention of preeclampsia with aspirin. American Journal of Obstetrics and Gynecology. 2022;**226**:S1108-S1119

[7] Walsh SW. Eicosanoids in preeclampsia. Prostaglandins, Leukotrienes, and Essential Fatty Acids. 2004;**70**:223-232

[8] Smith WL. The eicosanoids and their biochemical mechanisms of action. The Biochemical Journal. 1989;**259**:315-324

[9] Patrick J, Dillaha L, Armas D, et al. A randomized trial to assess the pharmacodynamics and pharmacokinetics of a single dose of an extended-release aspirin formulation. Postgraduate Medicine. 2015;**127**:573-580

[10] Walsh SW. Low-dose aspirin: Treatment for the imbalance of increased thromboxane and decreased prostacyclin in preeclampsia. American Journal of Perinatology. 1989;**6**:124-132

[11] Magee LA, Pels A, Helewa M, et al. Diagnosis, evaluation, and management of the hypertensive disorders of pregnancy: Executive summary. Journal of Obstetrics and Gynaecology Canada. 2014;**36**:416-438

[12] National institute for health and care excellence NICE. Hypertension in pregnancy: Diagnosis and management. NICE Guidelines. 2019;*NG133*:1-57

[13] Porter TF, Gyamfi-Bannerman C, Manuck T. ACOG Committee Opinion No. 743: Low-dose aspirin use during pregnancy. Obstetrics and Gynecology. 2018;**132**:E44-E52

[14] Villa PM, Kajantie E, Räikkönen K, et al. Aspirin in the prevention of pre-eclampsia in high-risk women: A randomised placebo-controlled PREDO trial and a meta-analysis of randomised trials. BJOG. 2013;**120**:64-74

[15] Rolnik DL, Wright D, Poon LCY, et al. ASPRE trial: Performance of screening for preterm pre-eclampsia. Ultrasound in Obstetrics & Gynecology. 2017;**50**:492-495

[16] Rogers MS, Fung HYM, Hung CY. Calcium and low-dose aspirin prophylaxis in women at high risk of pregnancy-induced hypertension. Hypertension in Pregnancy. 1999;**18**:165-172

[17] McParland P, Pearce JM, Chamberlain GVP. Doppler ultrasound and aspirin in recognition and prevention of pregnancy-induced hypertension. The Lancet. 1990;**335**:1552-1555

[18] Byaruhanga RN, Chipato T, Rusakaniko S. A randomized controlled trial of low-dose aspirin in women at risk from pre-eclampsia. International Journal of Gynecology & Obstetrics. 1998;**60**:129-135

[19] Tulppala M, Marttunen M, Söderström-Anttila V, et al. Low-dose aspirin in prevention of miscarriage in women with unexplained or autoimmune related recurrent miscarriage: Effect on prostacyclin and thromboxane A2 production. Human Reproduction. 1997;**12**:1567-1572

[20] Ayala DE, Ucieda R, Hermida RC. Chronotherapy with low-dose aspirin for prevention of complications in pregnancy. Chronobiology International. 2013;**30**:260-279

[21] CLASP: A randomised trial of low-dose aspirin for the prevention and treatment of pre-eclampsia among 9364 pregnant women. The Lancet. 1994;**343**:619-629

[22] Bujold E, Roberge S, Lacasse Y, et al. Prevention of preeclampsia and intrauterine growth restriction with aspirin started in early pregnancy: A meta-analysis. Obstetrics and Gynecology. 2010;**116**:402-414

[23] Roberge S, Villa P, Nicolaides K, et al. Early administration of low-dose aspirin for the prevention of preterm and term preeclampsia: A systematic review and meta-analysis. Fetal Diagnosis and Therapy. 2012;**31**:141-146

[24] Roberge S, Nicolaides K, Demers S, et al. The role of aspirin dose on the prevention of preeclampsia and fetal growth restriction: Systematic review and meta-analysis. American Journal of Obstetrics and Gynecology. 2017;**216**:110-120.e6

[25] Horgan R, Hage Diab Y, Waller J, Abuhamad A, Saade G. Low-dose aspirin therapy for the prevention of preeclampsia: Time to reconsider our recommendations? American Journal of Obstetrics and Gynecology. Oct 2023;**229**(4):410-418

[26] MacLennan AH, Thompson SC, Gecz J. Cerebral palsy: Causes, pathways, and the role of genetic variants. American Journal of Obstetrics and Gynecology. 2015;**213**:779-788

[27] Moore T, Hennessy EM, Myles J, Johnson SJ, Draper ES, Costeloe KL, et al. Neurological and developmental outcome in extremely preterm children born in England in 1995 and 2006: The EPICure studies. BMJ. 4 Dec 2012;**345**:e7961

[28] Oskoui M, Coutinho F, Dykeman J, et al. An update on the prevalence of cerebral palsy: A systematic review and meta-analysis. Developmental Medicine and Child Neurology. 2013;**55**:509-519

[29] Badawi N, Felix JF, Kurinczuk JJ, et al. Cerebral palsy following term newborn encephalopathy: A population-based study. Developmental Medicine and Child Neurology. 2005;**47**:293-298

[30] Chang E. Preterm birth and the role of neuroprotection. BMJ. 20 Jan 2015;**350**:g6661

[31] Kuban KC, Leviton A, Pagano M, et al. Maternal toxemia is associated with reduced incidence of germinal matrix hemorrhage in premature babies. Journal of Child Neurology. 1992;**7**:70-76

[32] Marret S, Marpeau L, Bénichou J. Benefit of magnesium sulfate given before very preterm birth to protect infant brain. Pediatrics. 2008;**121**:225-226

[33] Rouse DJ, Hirtz DG, Thom E, et al. A randomized, controlled trial of

magnesium sulfate for the prevention of cerebral palsy. The New England Journal of Medicine. 2008;**359**:895-905

[34] Mittendorf R, Dambrosia J, Pryde PG, et al. Association between the use of antenatal magnesium sulfate in preterm labor and adverse health outcomes in infants. American Journal of Obstetrics and Gynecology. 2002;**186**:1111-1118

[35] Crowther CA, Hiller JE, Doyle LW, et al. Effect of magnesium sulfate given for neuroprotection before preterm birth: A randomized controlled trial. JAMA. 2003;**290**:2669-2676

[36] Duley L, Farrell B, Armstrong N, et al. The magpie trial: A randomised trial comparing magnesium sulphate with placebo for pre-eclampsia. Outcome for children at 18 months. BJOG. 2007;**114**:289-299

[37] Doyle LW, Crowther CA, Middleton P, Marret S, Rouse D. Magnesium sulphate for women at risk of preterm birth for neuroprotection of the fetus. Cochrane Database of Systematic Reviews. 21 Jan 2009;**1**:CD004661

[38] Chollat C, Enser M, Houivet E, Provost D, Bénichou J, Marpeau L, et al. School-age outcomes following a randomized controlled trial of magnesium sulfate for neuroprotection of preterm infants. The Journal of Pediatrics. Aug 2014;**165**(2):398-400.e3

[39] Shepherd E, Salam RA, Middleton P, Makrides M, McIntyre S, Badawi N, et al. Antenatal and intrapartum interventions for preventing cerebral palsy: An overview of Cochrane systematic reviews. Cochrane Database of Systematic Reviews. 8 Aug 2017;**8**(8):CD012077

[40] Oddie S, Tuffnell DJ, McGuire W. Antenatal magnesium sulfate: Neuro-protection for preterm infants. Archives of Disease in Childhood. Fetal and Neonatal Edition. 2015;**100**:F553-F557

[41] Jayaram PM, Mohan MK, Farid I, et al. Antenatal magnesium sulfate for fetal neuroprotection: A critical appraisal and systematic review of clinical practice guidelines. Journal of Perinatal Medicine. 2019;**47**:262-269

[42] Roura LC i, Rodríguez DS, Rodríguez EC. Inducción a la madurez pulmonar. In: Obstetricia y medicina materno-fetal. 2007. ISBN 978-8-49-835594-9, 2007. pp. 255-262

[43] El-Sayed YY, Borders AEB. Gyamfi-Bannerman C. Committee opinion No. 713: Antenatal corticosteroid therapy for Fetal maturation. Obstetrics and Gynecology. 2017;**130**:E102-E109

[44] McGoldrick E, Stewart F, Parker R, Dalziel SR. Antenatal corticosteroids for accelerating fetal lung maturation for women at risk of preterm birth. Cochrane Database of Systematic Reviews. 25 Dec 2020;**12**(12):CD004454

[45] Harding JE, Pang JM, Knight DB, et al. Do antenatal corticosteroids help in the setting of preterm rupture of membranes? American Journal of Obstetrics and Gynecology. 2001;**184**:131-139

[46] Vidaeff AC, Ramin SM. Antenatal corticosteroids after preterm premature rupture of membranes. Clinical Obstetrics and Gynecology. 2011;**54**:337-343

[47] Brownfoot FC, Gagliardi DI, Bain E, Middleton P, Crowther CA. Different corticosteroids and regimens for accelerating fetal lung maturation for women at risk of preterm birth. Cochrane Database of Systematic Reviews. 29 Aug 2013;**8**:CD006764

[48] Ehsanipoor R. Practice bulletin No. 172: Premature rupture of membranes. Obstetrics and Gynecology. 2016;**128**:e165-e177

[49] Hayes EJ. Practice bulletin No. 169: Multifetal gestations: Twin, triplet, and higher-order multifetal pregnancies. Obstetrics and Gynecology. 2016;**128**:e131-e146

[50] Melamed N, Shah J, Yoon EW, Pelausa E, Lee SK, Shah PS, et al. The role of antenatal corticosteroids in twin pregnancies complicated by preterm birth. American Journal of Obstetrics and Gynecology. 2016;**215**(482):e1-482.e9

[51] Hay WW, Raju TN, Higgins RD, et al. Knowledge gaps and research needs for understanding and treating neonatal Hypoglycemia: Workshop Report from Eunice Kennedy Shriver National Institute of Child Health and Human Development. The Journal of Pediatrics. 2009;**155**:612-617

[52] Harris DL, Weston PJ, Harding JE. Incidence of neonatal hypoglycemia in babies identified as at risk. The Journal of Pediatrics. 2012;**161**:787-791

[53] Effect of corticosteroids for fetal maturation on perinatal outcomes, February 28—March 2, 1994. American Journal of Obstetrics and Gynecology. 1995;**173**:246-252

[54] Rubio EV, Socías P, Urquieta J, et al. Impact of prophylactic betamethasone indication on the neonatal outcome in 38-week pregnancies prior to elective Cesarean section. Open Journal of Obstetrics and Gynecology. 2020;**10**:1396-1401

[55] Crowther CA, Doyle LW, Haslam RR, et al. Outcomes at 2 years of age after repeat doses of antenatal corticosteroids. The New England Journal of Medicine. 2007;**357**:1179-1189

[56] Wapner RJ, Sorokin Y, Mele L, et al. Long-term outcomes after repeat doses of antenatal corticosteroids. The New England Journal of Medicine. 2007;**357**:1190-1198

[57] McKenna DS, Wittber GM, Nagaraja HN, et al. The effects of repeat doses of antenatal corticosteroids on maternal adrenal function. American Journal of Obstetrics and Gynecology. 2000;**183**:669-673

[58] Romero R, Conde-Agudelo A, El-Refaie W, et al. Vaginal progesterone decreases preterm birth and neonatal morbidity and mortality in women with a twin gestation and a short cervix: An updated meta-analysis of individual patient data. Ultrasound in Obstetrics & Gynecology. 2017;**49**:303-314

[59] Dodd JM, Jones L, Flenady V, Cincotta R, Crowther CA. Prenatal administration of progesterone for preventing preterm birth in women considered to be at risk of preterm birth. Cochrane Database of Systematic Reviews. 31 Jul 2013;7:CD004947

[60] Norman JE, Marlow N, Messow CM, et al. Vaginal progesterone prophylaxis for preterm birth (the OPPTIMUM study): A multicenter, randomised, double-blind trial. The Lancet. 2016;**387**:2106-2116

[61] Conde-Agudelo A, Romero R. Vaginal progesterone to prevent preterm birth in pregnant women with a sonographic short cervix: Clinical and public health implications. American Journal of Obstetrics and Gynecology. 2016;**214**:235-242

[62] Romero R, Conde-Agudelo A, Da Fonseca E, et al. Vaginal progesterone

for preventing preterm birth and adverse perinatal outcomes in singleton gestations with a short cervix: A meta-analysis of individual patient data. American Journal of Obstetrics and Gynecology. 2018;**218**:161-180

[63] Norman JE, Mackenzie F, Owen P, et al. Progesterone for the prevention of preterm birth in twin pregnancy (STOPPIT): A randomised, double-blind, placebo-controlled study and meta-analysis. Lancet. 2009;**373**:2034-2040

[64] Dodd JM, Grivell RM, OBrien CM, Dowswell T, Deussen AR. Prenatal administration of progestogens for preventing spontaneous preterm birth in women with a multiple pregnancy. Cochrane Database of Systematic Reviews. 20 Nov 2019;**2019**(11):CD012024